New NHS

A far-reaching programme of market-oriented changes has resulted in the emergence of a new National Health Service (NHS) where, increasingly, care is delivered by an 'alphabet soup' of agencies and public and private providers. Fundamental and complex changes have taken place in its structures and organisation, the system of funding and financing, governance and accountability. These are confusing, not only to the general public, but also to those working in healthcare, many of whom no longer have an understanding of the organisation they work for.

In this lucid and incisive account of the new NHS, Dr Alison Talbot-Smith, an experienced doctor and researcher, and Professor Allyson M. Pollock, one of the UK's leading authorities on the NHS, describe:

- the structures and functions of the new organisations, in each of the devolved countries
- the funding of NHS services, education, training and research and system of resource allocation, the regulation of the new NHS systems and workforce
- the new sets of relationships between the NHS, the Department of Health, local authorities and regulatory bodies, and between the NHS and the private sector
- the future implications of current policies.

This book will be invaluable to those working in healthcare today as clinicians, academics, researchers and managers. It will also be essential reading for academics, students and researchers in related fields, and for the general public, who need to understand the modern institutions of the NHS.

Dr Alison Talbot-Smith first trained in public health medicine, working for the NHS in London and researching at UCL. She has recently returned to clinical medicine as a specialist registrar in respiratory medicine.

Professor Allyson M. Pollock is head of the Centre for International Public Health Policy at the University of Edinburgh, honorary consultant in public health medicine at Lothian Health Board and Honorary Professor at UCL. She was, until recently, Director of Research and Development at UCL Hospitals NHS Foundation Trust and Head of the Public Health Policy unit at UCL. She trained in medicine in Scotland and public health in London.

The New NHS

A guide

**Alison Talbot-Smith and
Allyson M. Pollock
with Colin Leys and
Nick McNally**

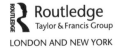
Routledge
Taylor & Francis Group

LONDON AND NEW YORK

First published 2006
by Routledge
2 Park Square, Milton Park, Abingdon, Oxon OX14 4RN

Simultaneously published in the USA and Canada
by Routledge
270 Madison Ave, New York, NY 10016

Routledge is an imprint of the Taylor & Francis Group, an informa business

© 2006 Alison Talbot-Smith and Allyson M. Pollock

Typeset in Times by
HWA Text and Data Management, Tunbridge Wells
Printed and bound in Great Britain by
MPG Books Ltd, Bodmin

British Library Cataloguing in Publication Data
A catalogue record for this book is available from the British Library

Library of Congress Cataloging-in-Publication Data
Talbot-Smith, Alison, 1968–
The new NHS : a guide / Alison Talbot-Smith and Allyson Pollock ; with Colin Leys and Nick McNally.
    p.   cm.
Includes bibliographical references and index.
1. National health services–Great Britain–Administration.
I. Pollock, Allyson. II. Leys, Colin. III. McNally, Nick. IV. Title.
[DNLM: 1. Great Britain. National Health Service. 2. State Medicine–organization & administration–Great Britain. W 225 FA1 T142n 2006]
RA395.G6T26 2006
362.1´0941–dc22   2005031143

ISBN10: 0–415–32841–1

ISBN13: 978–0–415–32841–8

Contents

Illustrations

Preface

The NHS is being radically transformed. It was originally conceived and built up as a tax-funded, centrally-planned, publicly-owned and accountable service, available everywhere to everyone equally, like schools or police services. The new NHS is to be a market, in which patients choose particular hospitals or clinics and in which doctors and hospitals compete for business, both with each other and with for-profit healthcare corporations.

This transition, involving quite drastic changes in almost every part of the service, is still in full swing, so that describing the emerging market-based system is tricky; things change before the ink is dry on the page – or before the text reaches hard copy. But the 1.3 million doctors, nurses, technicians, managers, and support staff of all kinds who already work in the NHS, and all those training for jobs in it, need to understand the emerging shape of the organization they work for, or hope to work for. So do social care professionals who interact closely with the NHS and suppliers who do business with it, as well as patients and their families, and many others. A guide is needed, even if, like other guides, it will need regular updating.

This is what *The New NHS* aims to provide: a guide which describes the emerging system accurately and clearly, with enough detail to be comprehensive, but not so much as to swamp the reader. There is a full table of contents and as good an index as we could make it. By definition the book focuses on the healthcare services provided by or for the NHS; social care services and long-term care for elderly people fall outside the remit of this book. For a discussion of this subject the reader could start by consulting Chapter 6 of Allyson Pollock, *NHS Plc: The Privatisation of our Health Care,* Verso, London, 2004.

Alison Talbot-Smith
Allyson Pollock
February 2006

Acknowledgements

We are grateful to Nick McNally, who wrote Chapter 7 of this book, and to Colin Leys for editing. We would also like to use this space to thank Virginia Hopson and James Lancaster, whose support and hard work were fundamental to its preparation and submission. Thanks are also due to those who provided information and comments, especially Sue Kerrison, Graham Petty, Catherine Brogan, Christine Hogg, Jon Ford, Ian Basnett, Jonathan Wise, Mark Hellowell and Jonathon Richards; and to staff at the British Medical Association and the Department of Health who kindly answered our many requests for information and data.

Abbreviations

AMCs	Academic Medical Centres
APMS	Alternative provider medical services
ARL	Annual resource limit
BMA	British Medical Association
BSA	Business Services Authority
CCI	Centre for Change and Innovation (Scotland)
CCT	Certificate of completion of training
CDO	Chief Dental Officer
CHAI	Commission for Healthcare Audit and Inspection
CHCs	Community Health Councils
CHI	Commission for Health Improvement
ChT	Children's trusts
CMO	Chief Medical Officer
COREC	Central Office for Research Ethics Committees
CPAG	Capital Prioritisation Advisory Group
CPPIH	Commission for Patient and Public Involvement in Health
CRDC	Central Research and Development Committee
CREST	Clinical Resource Efficiency Support Team
CRFF	Cancer Research Funders Forum
CRFs	Clinical Research Facilities
CRL	Capital resource limit
CSCI	Commission for Social Care Inspection
DH	Department of Health
DHA	District health authority
DHSS	Department of Health and Social Security
DHSSPS	Department of Health, Social Services and Public Safety (Northern Ireland)
DPH	Director of Public Health
DRGs	Diagnostic resource groups
DTC	Diagnostic and treatment centre
DTI	Department of Trade and Industry
FCE	Finished consultant episode
FT	Foundation trust

GDP	Gross domestic product
GDS	General dental services
GMC	General Medical Council
GMS	General medical services
GOS	General ophthalmic services
GP	General practitioner
HDA	Health Development Agency
HEFCE	Higher Education Funding Council for England
HES	Hospital episode statistics
HFEA	Human Fertilisation and Embryology Authority
HPA	Health Protection Agency
HPSS	Health and Personal Social Services (Northern Ireland)
HPU	Health protection unit (of the Health Protection Agency)
HRG	Health resource group
HSCIC	Health and Social Care Information Centre
ICAS	Independent Complaints Advocacy Service
ISTC	Independent sector treatment centre
IT	Information technology
KSF	Knowledge and skills framework
LDPs	Local Delivery Plans
LHB	Local health board (Wales)
LHCC	Local health care co-operative (Scotland)
LHSCG	Local health and social care group (Northern Ireland)
LIFT	Local improvement finance trust
LPS	Local pharmaceutical services
MHRA	Medicines and Healthcare Products Regulatory Agency
MRC	Medical Research Council
MRSA	Methicillin resistant staphylococcus aureus
NCAS	National Clinical Assessment Service
NCRI	National Cancer Research Institute
NCRN	National Cancer Research Network
NEAT	New and emerging applications of technology
NES	NHS Education for Scotland
NHS	National Health Service
NHS BT	NHS Blood and Transplant
NHS ILSI	NHS Institute for Learning, Skills and Innovation
NHS LIFT	NHS Local Improvement Finance Trust
NHSIA	NHS Information Authority
NHSLA	NHS Litigation Authority
NHSWD	NHS Wales Department (of Wales Assembly Government)
NICE	National Institute for Health and Clinical Excellence
NIMHE	National Institute for Mental Health
NPfIT	National Programme for Information Technology
NPSA	The National Patient Safety Agency
NRLS	National Reporting and Learning System

NSF	National Service Framework
NTA	National Treatment Agency for Substance Misuse
NTRAC	National Translational Cancer Research Network
NWCS	NHS wide clearing service
PALS	Patient Advice and Liaison Service
PASA	Purchasing and Supply Agency
PCT	Primary Care Trust
PCT MS	PCT medical services
PDP	Personal development plan
PDS	Personal dental services
PEC	Professional executive committee (of PCT)
PFI	Private finance initiative
PHO	Public health observatory
PICTF	Pharmaceutical Industry Competitiveness Taskforce
PMETB	The Postgraduate Medical Education and Training Board
PMS	Personal medical services
PNF	Priorities and needs funding
PPA	Prescription Pricing Authority
PPI forum	Patient and public involvement forum
QIS	Quality Improvement Scotland
QMAS	Quality management and analysis system
R&D	Research and development
RAFT	Regulatory Authority for Fertility and Tissue
RIA	Regulation Improvement Authority (Northern Ireland)
SDO	Service delivery and organisation
SEHD	Scottish Executive Health Department
SHA	Strategic health authority
SIFT	Service Increment for Teaching and Research
SIGN	Scottish Inter-Collegiate Guidelines Network
SLA	Service level agreement
SUS	Secondary uses services

1 Introduction

The NHS is in transition. Its publicly-funded system of publicly-owned and provided health care is being replaced by a healthcare market, in which public providers of services compete with private ones for NHS funds, with legal contracts and external regulation replacing direct political accountability. The pace of the transition is rapid, and the change is more far-reaching than is generally realised. The old structures and organisations are being dismantled and a plethora of new organisations and agencies is evolving.

In 1948 Aneurin Bevan famously promised that 'a dropped bed-pan would resound through the corridors of Whitehall', alluding to the strong system of political accountability which had been established. But just as steel bedpans have been replaced by disposable grey cardboard, the whole NHS has become in a sense disposable: its hundreds of hospitals and other organisations, transformed into independent market actors, must now increasingly fend for themselves financially. They are becoming answerable to market forces rather than elected ministers, and may even be closed down if they fail to give enough priority to solvency rather than patient care.*

For many if not most people within the NHS, not to mention those outside it, the new market-based relationships, and the array of new organisations and terminologies, are confusing. Many healthcare workers – doctors, nurses, paramedics, technical and ancillary staff, and even some administrators – no longer have a clear picture of how the NHS works, how its services are organised and accounted for, where its income comes from and how money flows through the system. Members of the general public are understandably even less clear. Yet understanding the way the NHS works has never been more important, and this book is intended to be a guide to the way it works now. The focus is unavoidably mainly on England, which as well as being the largest of the four countries of the UK is also the one where the drive to a healthcare market is most advanced; but a final chapter notes the most important ways in which Scotland, Wales and

---

* The official position of the Department of Health is that only 'non-essential' services will be allowed to close, but John Reid as Secretary of State stated that he personally would be prepared to see hospitals close (*Guardian* 3 February 2005). His successor Patricia Hewitt said she was ready to see 'services' close (*Guardian* 13 July 2005).

Northern Ireland, with their varying degrees of devolution, diverge from the English pattern.*

While the book aims to be descriptive rather than analytical, the significance of what it describes must not be lost sight of. So this chapter begins by setting out what the NHS was designed to do when it was first established in 1948, and how it evolved afterwards. It then briefly describes the transition to the market which began in the 1980s and was consolidated in 2000 by the NHS and Community Care Act of that year, and outlines the essential features of the new healthcare market.

The original NHS

The NHS was founded on three core principles. It was to be universal, i.e. to provide health care of the same standard throughout the UK. It was to be comprehensive, covering all health needs. And it was to be free at the point of delivery, available to all citizens equally on the basis of need, not ability to pay. To keep costs down, and to ensure efficiency and integration, the government abandoned the previous mixed system of social insurance (with employer and employee contributions) and private voluntary insurance, created by Lloyd George in 1911, in favour of central taxation. The insurance system had proved expensive and generated too much unfairness, leaving 50 per cent of the population, mainly women, children and older people, without coverage, and providing care of very uneven quality for those who were covered.

Funding

The arguments for using central taxation are compelling. Since 1948, successive governments have undertaken major reviews of the funding of the NHS – the most recent being that of Sir Derek Wanless in his final report for the Treasury in 2002 – and they have all concluded that central taxation remains the most efficient as well as the fairest system. First, central taxation is partly related to ability to pay. Second, it is cheaper to administer. Third, so long as there is also no internal invoicing and billing for treatments, it separates clinical decision-making from funding, allowing doctors to focus on what is best for each patient without any thought for the revenue they may represent. Fourth, and most fundamentally, it makes health care one of the things that binds society together, on the principle that we all take care of each other when things go wrong. Perhaps it was for this reason that, as ministers acknowledged in 1951, the NHS became 'the most popular of our new institutions' – a situation that has remained unchanged over six decades.[1]

---

* Where figures are given in this book they are generally for England, unless otherwise indicated.

There were also strong economic arguments for a centrally-administered system. Costs were kept low, partly because billing and marketing were eliminated, and partly because of the integrated nature of the system (what was a cost for one part of the NHS – money spent to prevent illnesses, for example – was a saving for other parts, in terms of primary care, hospitals, drugs, etc).

How the NHS's structures evolved from 1948 to 1980

From 1948 until 1980 the NHS evolved on the basis of rational planning, aimed at redistributing healthcare resources and services across the country on the basis of need and ensuring efficiency through integration. The aim was to make the health service as universally available and reliable as the postal service, and its structures were widely copied throughout the world.

Although the original NHS is often described as based on 'command and control' this is a mis-description, because despite the strong systems of bureaucracy and political accountability that were built into it much decision-making power was devolved to regional and district health authorities. Instructions were issued by the Department of Health (DH) but there was considerable local discretion to determine how local services were organised and delivered. Individual MPs and local authorities had a good deal of influence on local developments too – which sometimes worked for greater equity, and sometimes against it. And devolution for Scotland, Wales and Northern Ireland, introduced after 1997, allowed for still greater national autonomy and policy divergence.

The structures of the NHS were related to the nature of each kind of service it provided – preventative, primary, secondary and tertiary care.* The Department of Health and the NHS Executive were responsible for developing strategy and implementing policy, and for the performance of nationwide functions including workforce planning, managing the NHS's estates (its land and buildings), data collection and IT. In practice many of these functions were performed in conjunction with the regions and districts. Regional health authorities or (in Scotland and Northern Ireland) boards were responsible for planning and overseeing the

---

* Health services include prevention, primary care, secondary care and tertiary care. Preventative services include activities such as smoking cessation campaigns, but also interventions such as screening and immunisation. Primary care encompasses a range of services in the community including prevention, health promotion, GPs and health visitors and district nurses, paramedic services such as chiropody and dietetics, and services for people with mental health problems and learning disabilities. Secondary care describes a range of services usually provided in a hospital setting and includes inpatients, A and E, outpatients, diagnostics and pathology testing. Tertiary care refers to highly specialised care given in major hospital units to patients with rare, unusual or expensive conditions, involving expensive special equipment and tests. In addition there is a range of other specialist and support services including communicable disease control and public health and ambulance services which provide services across these tiers. These categories and groupings are changing rapidly, however. Treatments that used to be given in hospitals are now often provided by GPs, some surgery that used to require quite long hospital stays can now be done in day clinics, and so on.

provision of tertiary care in their regions and also for blood transfusion, cancer strategy and intensive care beds, IT, workforce strategy, ambulance services, training, and education. District health authorities were responsible for planning and providing secondary care (hospital) services for their local populations, and overseeing the provision of primary care. GPs were 'independent contractors' with the NHS, not directly employed by it, but there were strategies to bring about a more even distribution and supply of doctors and staff, including GPs, over time. Public health and communicable disease control were handled at all levels. In reality, planning was fluid and responsive to changing needs and circumstances, new technologies and advances.

Accountability and regulation

The NHS had a strong system of political accountability. All NHS organisations were directly accountable to the Secretary of State for Health through the DH. Detailed annual reports and accounts were laid before Parliament. There was also patient and public representation through the inclusion of local councillors and other members of the public on health authorities and boards. From 1974 onwards this was supplemented by Community Health Councils, local statutory independent bodies with some paid staff, but mainly made up of volunteers. NHS bodies were required to consult CHCs over any proposed major change in local services and CHCs could refer disputed changes to the Secretary of State.

The only areas where the state did not have the final word were in the regulation of the medical profession, and setting standards for training and accreditation. The medical professions regulated themselves. In the wake of the Nuremberg trials, which had highlighted the state-ordered wartime crimes of some German doctors, it was widely agreed that it was important to balance the role of the state in providing care with the freedom of the profession to practise to the highest independent ethical and professional standards. The General Medical Council or GMC, consisting of doctors from all specialties, was therefore responsible for certifying and licensing healthcare practitioners and for defining standards of education, clinical performance, and professional conduct to be followed by doctors. The GMC was supported by the Royal Colleges of medicine, professional organisations largely predating the NHS which set standards for education, training and knowledge in their respective fields. The DH had representation in the Colleges, but no authority to give them directions. Workforce planning was under the jurisdiction of the DH, since it controlled the number of places in medical schools, but at the postgraduate level the Colleges exercised considerable influence over the formation of specialists, being responsible for approving training places and training grades in NHS hospitals.

How money flowed through the system

In 1948 the NHS inherited an inequitable distribution of services, and critics pointed to the fact that resources still flowed to where they had always been more plentiful, rather than areas of greatest need. To remedy this the government eventually appointed a resource allocation working party (RAWP) which led to the establishment of a fairer system whereby revenue for hospital and community health services was distributed on the basis of resident population size, adjusted for indicators of the local need for services and the local costs of providing them. True equity was still far from being achieved, but the distribution of resources did gradually become more even throughout the country.

Hospitals received annual budgets from the health authorities. Revenue for primary care services was distributed to individual GPs on the basis of the numbers of patients on their lists, supplemented by a system of fees and allowances to cover their infrastructure (surgeries and equipment), as well as for achieving targets such as immunisation rates.

The transition to a market

The transition to a market has occurred over several decades, the result of more than 30 acts of Parliament. The consensus that the NHS should be under public ownership and control was gradually undermined by disagreement over levels of funding for the NHS, what it should and could provide, and how it could be run efficiently – and by the effects of chronic under-funding, which had dogged it from its inception, leading to long waiting times and dilapidated premises. It was of course also the target of a great deal of hostile commentary in the media, focussing exclusively on its shortcomings – which were real enough in practice, as they are in any complex public or private service – even though the level of public support for the NHS remained remarkably constant.

The 1980s: general management and outsourcing

A decisive turning-point was reached in 1979, when Mrs Thatcher came to power. The Thatcher administration quickly introduced two new policies of great long-term significance: general management, and the outsourcing or 'contracting out' of non-clinical services such as hospital cleaning, laundry and catering. General management introduced a new layer of hospital managers, increasingly trained and disciplined in business methods, between the civil service and healthcare professionals, distancing policy-makers from the doctor–patient interface; while outsourcing catering and cleaning services introduced the private sector for the first time directly into the provision of NHS care. The outsourced services were turned into very profitable businesses, some of which were floated on the stock market.

Long-term residential care for frail elderly or disabled people also began to be privatised under the Thatcher governments.* By the end of the 1990s free long-

---

* As already mentioned in the Preface, this book does not deal with long-term care, only a very small portion of which is now provided by the NHS. For an account of its transfer out of the NHS see Chapter 6 of Pollock, A. (2004), *NHS Plc: The Privatisation of Our Health Care*, London: Verso, second edition.

term care provided by the NHS had been largely replaced by care in independent sector care homes (mainly for-profit), for which fees had to be paid.

The 1990s: the 'internal market' and the Private Finance Initiative

In 1991 the government restructured the NHS more radically, creating a so-called 'internal market'. The 1990 NHS and Community Care Act turned NHS hospitals, or groups of hospitals, and other bodies like ambulance and community health services, into semi-independent 'trusts', and required them to behave like businesses in a marketplace. The health authorities became 'commissioners' or 'purchasers' of health services, and the trusts became 'sellers'. Although the 'contracts' involved in these transactions had no legal force, the DH required them to be honoured, and the new system brought about a sea-change in the way NHS resources and the funding of services were accounted for.

The provision of services was still meant to be based on an assessment of the needs for services in each area, but since NHS hospitals and other services could no longer rely on an annual block budget they no longer had an incentive to give priority to needs. They now had to break even by generating their own income and cutting costs, and competing with each other for business. The priority became what would allow them to balance the books.

All of these measures were aimed at increasing efficiency and choice, but hospitals and community services which were already short of resources now faced the extra costs involved in competing for funding, dealing with risk, and administering the complexities of making and monitoring hundreds of contracts. Within a short space of time more than a third of the new trusts faced serious financial difficulties and were forced into mergers and service closures (between 1990 and 1994, 245 hospitals were closed in England and Wales).

Another change was that trusts were no longer given free support from the DH's regional offices for capital planning, estates management and IT. In the interest of business efficiency they now had to buy these services from private management consultancies out of the revenue they earned from the services they 'sold'. The resources and expertise of the NHS regional offices in these areas were disbanded.

The introduction of the 'internal market' also changed the way in which NHS capital was accounted for. For the first time all NHS service providers – now constituted as semi-independent trusts – had to pay an annual charge (originally 6 per cent) on the value of their land and equipment, out of the revenue they 'earned'. Known as the 'capital charge', it was paid to the Treasury. The idea was to make trusts more economical with their capital assets – and to encourage them to sell off any they did not need, or which were too valuable (such as land in city centres) – by making them pay for their use.

But capital charging also paved the way for a more profound change, the Private Finance Initiative or PFI. The PFI was introduced by the government in 1992 as an alternative way of mobilising capital for public investments. A consortium of bankers, construction companies and 'facilities management' firms come together in a joint venture to design, build and operate NHS premises in return for an annual charge paid by the NHS over the life-time of a contract, usually 25–30 years. In effect NHS trusts lease back their facilities, paying an annual fee to the PFI consortium instead of a capital charge to the Treasury. In reality these leases are often extended more or less indefinitely through the renegotiation of contracts. By 2005, 50 hospital building schemes, out of the 100 promised in 2000 in *The NHS Plan*, were operational, 42 of them via the PFI;[2] and the total value of PFI-financed hospital schemes approved since 1997 was £17 billion, creating a very large new business sector closely tied into the provision of NHS clinical services.[3]

Meantime a further step was taken towards a full market when the purchasing was devolved from district health authorities to some 300 'Primary Care Trusts' or PCTs, each representing the local primary care community (GPs, dentists, etc.) and local residents. By the early 2000s 80 per cent of the total NHS budget was being distributed to PCTs, which now 'commission' all NHS secondary (hospital) care as well as primary care.

The emerging market in clinical care

Until 2000 the government maintained that clinical services would not be privatised, but *The NHS Plan*, published in 2000, made it clear that they would after all be opened up to the market, in order to provide much-needed additional capacity.[3] It quickly became apparent, however, that private providers could not provide significant volumes of services without using NHS doctors and staff, and the policy rationale shifted from providing extra capacity to giving patients a wider choice of service providers.

The model that gradually emerged from a succession of policy statements was thus of the NHS as a sort of holding company, 'franchising' health services out to various providers, public and private. The NHS is to be the government-funded payer, but less and less the direct provider, of health services. The old system based on political accountability (and on public trust in the service ethos of the NHS workforce) is giving way to one based on private law and legally binding contracts. With this shift comes a new way of setting and enforcing standards via monitoring, inspections, auditing and legal challenges. This means new organisations and regulatory bodies. A market also means new costs: the costs of 'marketing' services to attract patients, billing and invoicing, fees for management consultancies and lawyers and, for private sector providers of NHS services, the payment of dividends. A much-simplified outline of the shape of the new NHS can be seen in Figure 1.1.

The structures and relationships of the new market

The shift to market forces in place of Parliament as the prime determinant of what health services are offered has led to radical changes in the structure of the NHS,

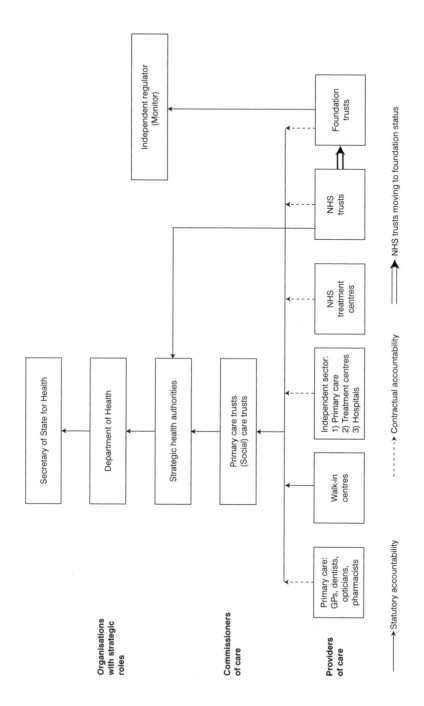

Figure 1.1 The structure of the new NHS in England

starting at the top. The Department of Health is being 'downsized' by almost 40 per cent of its staff, as its functions are progressively transferred to the market. Perhaps its main remaining strategic role is to set the prices at which services are sold in the new healthcare market, in a so-called 'national tariff'. By the end of the decade all NHS trusts' services are to be paid for on the basis of 'payment by results', i.e. a payment for every treatment given; but they will not be allowed to compete by cutting prices for any of their services; prices are to be set for every treatment or procedure. So long as price competition continues to be ruled out, the prices set in the national tariff will be crucial in determining whether providers make a surplus or a loss by agreeing to provide the particular mix and volume of services that the local purchasers (now called 'commissioners') want. Some treatments are likely to prove profitable, and others not, and providers will inevitably want to do more of the former and fewer of the latter. If this is not to lead to services being unavailable for some patients who need the less profitable treatments, the prices will have to be constantly adjusted, a task that would appear to call for a lot of information and – in effect – expertise in the much-maligned business of planning, which the DH will have to maintain at a high enough level for this purpose.

Regulating the market

Apart from this, however – and managing the important international trade aspects of healthcare provision, as the NHS is opened up to what is an increasingly international market of healthcare providers – the DH is fast assuming a much more restricted role, 'steering not rowing' (to use the government's expression). NHS hospitals, ambulances, community care trusts, etc. will be regulated by two new 'arm's length' bodies (i.e. at arm's length from the DH): the Healthcare Commission, and the independent regulator, Monitor.

The Healthcare Commission supervises and inspects (and in the case of private and voluntary healthcare providers, licenses) all providers of secondary and tertiary care. It also 'rates' all NHS trusts on what used to be called a 'star' system (the terminology of three, two, one or no 'stars' has been abandoned, but not the rating system or the 'league tables' it produces). How well trusts do in these annual ratings determines the pace at which they are allowed to move towards 'foundation' status. Foundation trusts (FTs) are trusts that have been judged ready to fend entirely for themselves in the new healthcare market, without support from the DH. This judgment is made by Monitor, the office of the independent regulator. Once granted FT status, trusts cease to be subject to supervision by the local Strategic Health Authority (SHA), and are supervised purely by Monitor, with input from the Healthcare Commission.

Monitor is concerned above all with FTs' financial viability. While it asks whether they are serving the health needs of the local population, the only indicator of this that is explicitly taken into account is whether the PCTs commissioning their services are satisfied. The financial viability of foundation trusts depends on how far they can 'generate' income (including income they may generate from joint ventures with private companies, which need not have anything to do with health care) and reduce costs; and on the way they use their freedoms to borrow on the private financial markets, sell assets, outsource clinical activities, etc.

In the meantime, however, the performance of NHS trusts which have not yet been granted foundation status (still the great majority) is managed by the DH's 28 Strategic Health Authorities or SHAs. SHAs supervise all aspects of NHS trusts' operations, and especially the extent to which they are achieving all the government's national targets and standards. But all NHS trusts – including, perhaps, PCTs – are expected to become FTs by the end of the decade, so SHAs seem likely to be transitional organisations. The future regulation of the NHS will then lie largely in the hands of the Healthcare Commission and Monitor.

Professional self-regulation is also giving way to more external regulation. The role of the Royal Colleges has been significantly reduced; standards of care will increasingly be determined by the Healthcare Commission (through its inspections) and Monitor through its licensing, and by 'National Service Frameworks' (essentially protocols setting out standard procedures to be followed for specific medical conditions); while the government-appointed 'deaneries', which administer postgraduate medical training policy, are shortening the period of specialist training. The GMC is also being remodelled, reducing the professional element in it, while new contracts for both GPs and consultants give the government (and will eventually give the private sector) considerable powers to determine how doctors work. How far patients' interests will still come first under these conditions remains to be seen.

Restructuring the workforce

The shift to a market also called for important changes in the terms of service of NHS staff, to introduce the labour market 'flexibility' that responding to market pressures is seen as requiring. Flexible conditions for ancillary staff were introduced in 2003 in an initiative called 'Agenda for Change', and new contracts for hospital consultants and GPs were negotiated at the same time. The new consultants' contract allows FTs to vary their conditions of service, and to direct them to work in the private sector if trust policy involves outsourcing work, or for other reasons. The new GPs' contract ended GPs' longstanding monopoly over the provision of primary care and opened it up to corporate providers.

*****

The following Chapters 2 to 9 describe the NHS as it is today – its main organisations and how they relate to each other, how it is funded and regulated, how it funds and regulates research, the scale and skills of its workforce, and the main ways in which devolution has confirmed, and in some cases accentuated, differences between the way the NHS works in England, Scotland, Wales and Northern Ireland. These chapters have only one aim: to describe the new NHS as clearly as possible, with a minimum of jargon and just enough concrete detail to make its complexities easier to grasp. A very brief final chapter (Chapter 10) moves from description to questions, suggesting some of the issues that are at stake as the new market-based NHS becomes fully operational.

2 Organisations with strategic roles

This chapter describes organisations whose role is primarily strategic, determining the overall direction of the NHS in England, and overseeing and co-ordinating the work of other NHS organisations. Ultimate responsibility for the NHS lies with Parliament, through the Secretary of State for Health, whose Department of Health is in turn supported by various 'arm's length bodies' – organisations which provide specific national functions on its behalf. At the regional level, implementing NHS strategy is the responsibility of Strategic Health Authorities (SHAs).

At the parliamentary level, in addition to the Secretary of State there are five junior ministers with responsibility for various aspects of the NHS: two ministers of state and three parliamentary under-secretaries (Table 2.1).

The Department of Health

Functions

With offices in London and Leeds the Department of Health (DH) is responsible for both health and social services, with the overall aim of improving the health and well-being of the people of England (Box 2.1). It advises government ministers on health and healthcare issues and sets out the national policy determined by them. It is directly responsible for providing health services via the NHS. It does not 'run' the NHS but it sets national policy, provides advice and guidance, and oversees the performance of NHS organisations. With respect to social care services the DH sets out ministerial policy and provides advice and guidance to the local authorities which provide the services.

In conjunction with the reform and re-organisation of the NHS, the DH has itself been re-organised to assume a more purely strategic role: responsibility for NHS service delivery is being increasingly devolved to 'frontline' organisations, especially Primary Care Trusts (PCTs) and NHS hospital trusts. Responsibility for managing, inspecting and regulating services is also being increasingly devolved to Strategic Health Authorities, 'arm's length bodies', and other organisations; for example the Healthcare Commission and the independent regulator of NHS foundation trusts, Monitor, are now responsible for inspecting and assessing the performance of NHS organisations and foundation trusts respectively, while

Table 2.1 Ministerial responsibilities for the NHS, January 2006

Secretary of State for Health	Patricia Hewett	Responsible for the work of the Department of Health, in particular NHS service delivery and reform; finance and resources; media and communications
Minister of State for NHS Delivery	Lord Warner	NHS finance and workforce issues (including education and pay); primary care; chronic disease; access and delivery (including emergency care); information technology; NHS foundation trusts; the private finance initiative; LIFT; and patient choice
Minister of State for Health Services	Rosie Winterton	Specific services (cancer, cardiac, diabetes, mental health, renal, prison, dentistry); emergency preparedness; equality and diversity; patient and public involvement; international issues
Minister of State for Quality and Patient Safety	Jane Kennedy	NHS standards, inspection, and performance; patient safety; clinical governance and quality issues (e.g. NICE and MRSA); clinical negligence; research and development; pharmaceutical industry and regulation of medicines and healthcare products; departmental management
Parliamentary Under-Secretary for Public Health	Caroline Flint	Preventative services (e.g. activity and nutrition); communicable diseases and sexual health; health inequalities; drugs, tobacco and alcohol; sustainable development; food standards agency; human fertilisation and embryology authority
Parliamentary Under-Secretary of State for Care Services	Liam Byrne	Finance, performance, inspection, and workforce for social care services; children's health; maternity services; mental health and older people's services; physical and learning disabilities services; services provided by allied health professionals and the voluntary sector

Source: Department of Health website.

Box 2.1   Aims and objectives of the Department of Health

Aims

To improve the health and well being of the people of England by:

• Supporting activity at national level to protect, promote and improve the nations health

• Securing the provision of comprehensive, high quality care for all those who need it, regardless of their ability to pay or where they live or their age

• Securing responsive social care and child protection for those who lack the support they need

Objectives

The key objectives in pursuing these aims are:

• To reduce the incidence of avoidable illness, disease and injury in the population

• To treat people with illness, disease or injury quickly, effectively and on the basis of need alone

• To enable people, who are unable to perform essential activities of daily living, including those with chronic illness, disability or terminal illness, to live as full and normal lives as possible

• To maximise the social development of children within stable family settings

• To assure performance and support to Ministers in accounting to Parliament and the public for the overall performance of the NHS, personal social services and the Department of Health

• To manage the resources and staff of the Department of Health so as to improve performance

Source: Department of Health (2004), *Departmental Report 2004*, London

---

responsibility for the day-to-day negotiation of pay and conditions of service issues has been transferred to NHS Employers, an organisation set up by the NHS Confederation of Managers.

The core functions of the DH are essentially threefold. First, to secure and distribute resources – in 2004 the department was responsible for £78 billion of public funds[1] – and make major investment decisions. Second, to set national strategy and the 'overall direction' for the NHS and social care. This currently includes extending patients' ability to choose their service providers and ensuring that national standards based on solid research evidence are set and maintained. Third, to account to Parliament for the overall performance of the

NHS, but operating at 'arm's length' from the day-to-day work of successful NHS organisations and intervening only where necessary.

Structure

The DH's gross administrative costs were estimated at £306 million for the year 2003–4, when it employed 3,350 staff.[2] In October 2004, however, it was re-structured, reducing its size by 38 per cent to 2,272 staff.[3] As a corporate body (i.e. one whose work is led and overseen by a board of directors) it is now headed by a Management Board, which oversees the work of three business groups (Figure 2.1).

The Management Board is chaired by the Chief Executive of the NHS, who since 2000 has also been the Permanent Secretary of the DH. It has seven directors, drawn from the three business groups, although the intention is also to include non-executive directors drawn from local government and the private sector.[4] The board is responsible for the overall direction of the DH and for overseeing corporate governance (the internal management arrangements of the organisation). The three business groups cover the work areas described below.

The Health and Social Care Standards and Quality Group

This group is led by the Chief Medical Officer for England. As the major policy-making body it is responsible for overseeing the standards and quality of health and social care services, as well as maintaining and promoting health and well-being, protecting the population's health, and ensuring the safety of patients. It sets standards and defines quality for health and social services, as well as promoting public health through policies addressing issues such as healthier lifestyles and inequalities in health. It oversees the work of the Health Protection Agency (see ppp. 75–7), which is responsible for communicable disease control and environmental health issues. It is also responsible for research and development, and for achieving the aims of government programmes such as improving the prevention and treatment of coronary heart disease and cancer. It is thus responsible for setting policy in a very diverse range of areas, from lifestyle issues such as smoking and obesity to scientific and technical innovations such as stem-cell research.

The Health and Social Care Delivery Group

This group is responsible for the delivery of NHS services. Its remit encompasses finance and investment: the group is responsible for securing resources from the Treasury for both NHS and local authority (social care) services as well as overseeing the financial performance of NHS organisations. It is also responsible for 'performance and service improvement', securing delivery of the government's priorities in health and social care set out as targets in the 2000 publication, *The NHS Plan*. This includes the work of a new Commercial Directorate, headed by a senior businessman, responsible for promoting the adoption of commercial

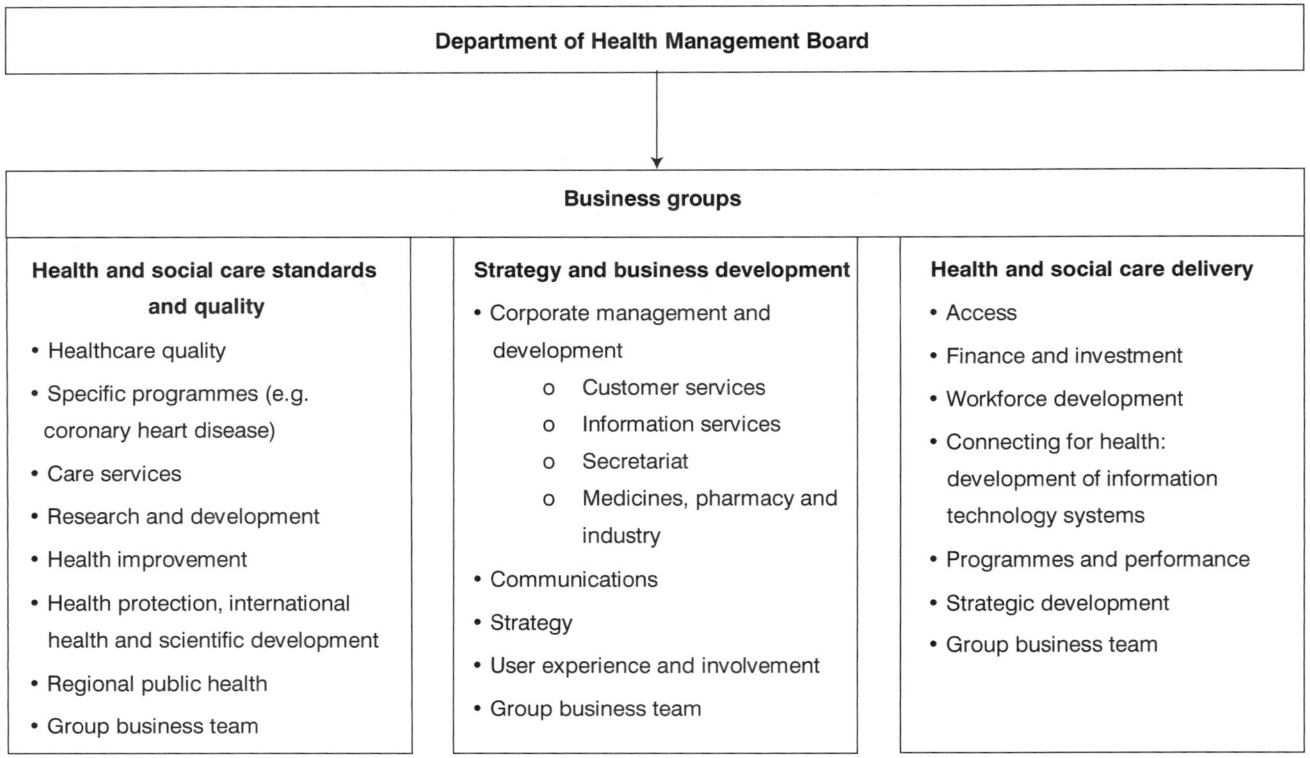

Department of Health Management Board

Business groups

Health and social care standards and quality

- Healthcare quality
- Specific programmes (e.g. coronary heart disease)
- Care services
- Research and development
- Health improvement
- Health protection, international health and scientific development
- Regional public health
- Group business team

Strategy and business development

- Corporate management and development
  - o Customer services
  - o Information services
  - o Secretariat
  - o Medicines, pharmacy and industry
- Communications
- Strategy
- User experience and involvement
- Group business team

Health and social care delivery

- Access
- Finance and investment
- Workforce development
- Connecting for health: development of information technology systems
- Programmes and performance
- Strategic development
- Group business team

Figure 2.1 The structure of the Department of Health, 2005

practices throughout the NHS; and for 'smart procurement' from, and developing links with, the private sector, which as Chapter 1 explains is of fast-growing importance in the new NHS.

The Group is also in charge of developing the NHS workforce, increasing the capacity of NHS services, enabling patients to have a choice of hospitals, and achieving 'access' targets such as shorter waiting times for primary care and hospital appointments. As part of this remit the Group is responsible for 'performance managing' the Strategic Health Authorities or SHAs in terms of their management capacity, financial balance, and the performance of the NHS in their areas. This work is undertaken through meetings with SHA chief executives and through annual appraisals against a 'performance assessment framework', discussed more fully in Chapter 6 (pages 108–9). The Group is also responsible for delivery of the 'National Programme for Information Technology' (discussed below, page 23), which is intended to provide an integrated information and technology system throughout the NHS.

The Strategy and Business Development Group

This group is responsible for 'corporate' services, such as human resources, customer services, and DH communications. It also sets policy on specific programmes such as user involvement and experience, and medicines and pharmacy development, and includes a recently-created Strategy Directorate to support the Management Board and DH ministers in setting goals and policy objectives.

Supporting activities within the Department of Health

The work of the DH Management Board and business groups is supported by a number of other appointments and work areas within the Department. These include the 'heads of profession', who provide expert knowledge in specialist health and social care disciplines.* There are also nine 'national clinical directors', clinicians who provide advice and leadership on implementing the DH's national clinical priorities.†

An 'NHS Modernisation Board' also supports the work of the DH by overseeing the implementation of the *NHS Plan*. It monitors progress made by the DH, the NHS, local authorities and other members of the social care community, such as voluntary agencies, against the commitments and targets in the Plan. It also advises on how obstacles to change can be overcome, and seeks to facilitate dialogue between the DH, the NHS, and patients.

* The heads of profession are the Chief Medical Officer, the Chief Nursing Officer, the Chief Dental Officer, the Chief [allied] Health Professions Officer, the Chief Scientific Officer, the Chief Pharmaceutical Officer and the Chief Inspector of the Commission for Social Care Inspection.
† These priorities are: emergency access; mental health; children's services; heart disease; primary care; older people's services; cancer; diabetes; patient and public involvement (non-clinician).

The Modernisation Board was announced in *The NHS Plan* and established in April 2001. It is chaired by the Secretary of State for Health, who also appoints its 35 members.[5] Although they are appointed in their individual capacities they are drawn from senior managerial and clinical members of health and social care organisations (especially NHS trusts and PCTs), the Royal Colleges, trade unions (the British Medical Association and Unison), local government, the NHS Confederation [of managers], private healthcare organisations (such as General Healthcare Group), voluntary organisations and patient support groups. The Board meets quarterly with the Secretary of State, as well as reporting directly to Parliament and publishing an annual report detailing progress made in achieving *NHS Plan* targets.

Strategic Health Authorities (SHAs)

SHAs are the regional bodies responsible for ensuring that DH strategic policies are followed by the NHS bodies which commission ('purchase') or provide health services throughout England (different organisations do this work in Wales and Northern Ireland, and commissioning has been abolished in Scotland – see Chapter 9).

Establishment

Twenty-eight SHAs were established in April 2002 and became fully operational in October of that year.* Each covers an average population of 1.5 million,[6] with boundaries corresponding to the outer boundaries of groups of local authorities. They vary considerably in geographic scope – for example five SHAs cover London, while Cheshire and Merseyside SHA alone covers over 1,000 square miles and a population of around 2.4 million.[7] At the time of writing, however, the DH had indicated its intention to reduce the number of SHAs, to make them larger organisations covering larger populations. The reduction suggested was from 28 to nine SHAs, with boundaries generally in alignment with those of the Government Offices of the Regions. Actual reconfigurations are to be determined through a process led by SHAs themselves; the DH intends that the new boundaries be in place by April 2007.

When first introduced SHAs were described as being under three-year 'franchises'; candidate chief executives applied to the DH for their positions, and selected applicants had to prepare three year 'franchise plans', detailing how the SHA in question would achieve its assigned goals. The plans included proposals for the structure and competencies of the management team and formed the basis of performance clauses in their senior management contracts. However there seems to have been a move away from the 'franchise' approach, with franchise plans replaced by SHA Local Delivery Plans which spell out the planned health

---

*   Prior to April 2002 there were 100 district health authorities, overseen by four regional 'outposts' of the DH known as directorates of health and social care.

and service delivery improvements to be achieved in the next three years by the whole 'local health economy'.

SHAs may, however, have a limited lifespan. If all NHS trusts and ultimately PCTs achieve foundation status (as described in Chapter 4, pages 63–6) they will fall outside the jurisdiction of SHAs, most of whose present functions will then lapse.

Function

The SHAs' function is strategic; they are the link between the strategically-focused DH and the 'frontline' operations of PCTs and NHS hospital trusts. Often described as the 'local headquarters' of the NHS, they are responsible for overseeing the day-to-day management of the NHS in their areas, each SHA having an average of some 25 organisations to oversee.[8] These include PCTs as well as a variety of NHS trusts, ranging from acute hospital trusts and specialist trusts providing specific services such as orthopaedics or learning disability services, to mental health trusts and ambulance trusts.

SHAs have three main responsibilities. The first is to create a coherent strategic framework for the local development of services; this is in effect a responsibility for overseeing the planning and development of healthcare services in their areas. It involves bringing together the Local Delivery Plans of primary care trusts and the business plans of NHS trusts, to produce a Local Delivery Plan for the whole SHA area which details planned health and service improvements over the next three years.

The second responsibility is to build the capacity of local services. This involves developing strategies for capital investment and overseeing investments as they are made, allocating funds for 'strategic' capital development (see Chapter 5, page 89), and approving the business cases of major capital development schemes put forward by PCTs and other NHS trusts. It also involves overseeing information management, such as co-ordinating the implementation of the National Programme for Information Technology (NPfIT – see below page 23). Workforce development is also included here, overseeing the allocation of funds for new posts, co-ordinating PCTs' and NHS trusts' resources for workforce development, and giving training in leadership skills to consultants, clinical directors and senior executives, as well as providing education and development programmes for the local NHS workforce.

The third responsibility is 'performance managing' the NHS organisations in their area, other than foundation trusts: namely PCTs, NHS hospital trusts, and other trusts such as care trusts and mental health trusts. This involves overseeing their performance on the basis of annual 'accountability agreements' made between each PCT or NHS trust chief executive and a nominated SHA director. The latter holds the PCTs and NHS trusts to account for achieving financial balance, and for their achievement of the agreed performance targets laid out in their Local Delivery Plans (for PCTs) or business plans (for NHS trusts). These agreements address national (NHS Plan) priorities, including targets for access to services and waiting time in accident and emergency, local priorities such as immunisation rates, and organisational and workforce development issues such as GP appraisals. Performance is monitored throughout the year by the SHA performance management team, through meetings with PCT or NHS trust performance managers, as well as by monitoring weekly, monthly and quarterly returns (submissions by Primary Care trusts and NHS trusts which detail levels of activity and performance). More formal accountability meetings are held at least annually with trust chairs and chief executives, at frequencies that depend upon the performance of the PCT or NHS trust (i.e. less frequently for well-performing organisations).

Structure

SHAs are corporate bodies whose work is overseen by boards consisting of both executive and non-executive members. The board is responsible for overseeing the strategic direction of the SHA, providing stewardship of its assets and finances, ensuring that it delivers its agreed objectives and that systems are in place for the delivery of quality services. SHAs have relative freedom to determine the structure of their boards; although they must include the chief executive and the director of finance, they may also have up to five executive directors and up to seven non-executive members (appointed by the NHS Appointments Commission – see below, pages 31–2).

The senior management team is responsible for overseeing the day-to-day functioning of the SHA, and achieving the aims and objectives determined by the board. SHAs have some freedom to determine their working arrangements, such as the structure and functions of their senior management teams, although the team must always include a public health doctor or a medical director. There is a cap on SHA staffing numbers of 75, although many SHAs are smaller than this, particularly in areas such as London where office rents are high. There is also a cap on their annual management costs (£4 million each in 2005). Given these constraints, SHAs cannot address all aspects of their remit equally. In many if not most SHAs, the performance management team is the largest staffing element.

'Arm's length' bodies of the Department of Health

The DH is also supported in its work by a number of 'arm's length bodies'. These are distinct from the numerous advisory bodies which assist the DH in developing and evaluating policy: arm's length bodies are organisations funded by the DH to undertake particular functions on its behalf, such as business, procurement and regulatory functions.Their staff must follow prescribed codes of practice and declare any relevant interests. Where appropriate open meetings must be held and summary reports published. They are accountable to the DH and sometimes also to Parliament. They are of three types: DH executive agencies, special health authorities, and non-departmental public bodies.

In 2003–4, 38 such bodies existed or were planned. Between them they employed 25,000 staff, with total annual operating costs of £1.8 billion and annual expenditure on services totalling £3 billion. Following a review published in July 2004 the number of arm's length bodies will be reduced to 19 by 2007–8, with the aim of reducing staff numbers by 25 per cent and operating costs by at least £500 million.[9] The DH is also exploring the possibility of devolving funding to the local level, so that local NHS organisations would 'buy' services from the arm's length bodies, which would then 'earn' their funding in this way.

The 19 arm's length bodies intended to be in operation by 2007–8 are discussed here – three executive agencies of the DH, eight special health authorities, and eight non-departmental public bodies (see Table 2.2). For bodies not yet or only recently in operation at the time of writing, both their intended functions and the functions of their constituent organisations are discussed.*

Executive agencies of the DH

Executive agencies are self-contained units of the DH. Rather than giving policy advice they carry out specific 'executive' functions on behalf of the DH. They function independently from the DH but are funded by and accountable to it.

The NHS Purchasing and Supply Agency (PASA)

This agency was launched in April 2000. With 318 staff in 2003–4 its operating costs were £20.8 million.[10] It is a co-ordinating and advisory body on purchasing and supply issues, negotiating contracts for goods and services on behalf of the NHS, providing advice to individual NHS organisations (for example regarding the best choice of device for a particular purpose), developing electronic ordering systems and holding a data-base of NHS suppliers. It also gives training to NHS purchasing staff, providing 2,000 training places in 2003.[11]

The Purchasing and Supply Agency acts as a centre of excellence for purchasing and supply matters within the NHS; the intention is that by 2007–8 it should deliver annual savings to the NHS of £280 million.[12] The agency will also begin to commission services such as pensions services on behalf of the NHS from a

---

* One formerly important executive agency, NHS Estates, was privatised in April 2005. With 218 staff and operating costs of £29.5 million in 2003–4 its role was to enable a modern environment for patient care. Its 'policy and performance management' team provided support and advice to NHS organisations on the procurement, design, operation and maintenance of healthcare buildings and facilities. It also had a trading arm, a public–private partnership called 'Inventures' which carried out activities such as the disposal of NHS estate. A 'core' team was taken from NHS Estates into the DH, but Inventures, with an annual turnover of £40 million and £400 million of (NHS) property and land assets, was sold to a private consortium (Miller Ventures and Construction).

Table 2.2   Arm's length bodies of the Department of Health by mid-2008.

Executive agencies of the Department of Health
NHS Purchasing and Supply Agency
Medicine and Healthcare Products Regulatory Agency
National Programme for Information Technology
Special health authorities
NHS Institute for Learning Skills and Innovation
Business Services Authority
NHS Litigation Authority
Health and Social Care Information Centre
National Patient Safety Agency
National Institute for Health and Clinical Excellence
National Treatment Agency for Substance Misuse
NHS Blood and Transplant
Executive non-departmental public bodies
Monitor (the independent regulator of NHS foundation trusts)
Commission for Healthcare Audit and Inspection (the Healthcare Commission)
Council for the Regulation of Healthcare Professionals
Health Protection Agency
NHS Appointments Commission
Regulatory Authority for Fertility and Tissue
Postgraduate Medical Education and Training Board
General Social Care Council

Source: Department of Health, An implementation framework for reconfiguring the DH arm's length bodies, 2004.

new NHS Business Services Authority (see below), and healthcare products and supply-chain services from a privatised NHS Logistics Authority.[*]

The Medicine and Healthcare Products Regulatory Agency (MHRA)

This agency became operational in April 2003, following a merger of the Medical Devices Agency with the Medicines Control Agency. Its role is to

---

[*]   The NHS Logistics Authority was a special health authority established in April 2000 to provide consumable healthcare products and supply-chain services to NHS trusts in order to improve the efficiency with which products were supplied to the NHS. Stocking over 40,000 lines of healthcare products it also had an electronic ordering service known as Logistics On-line. In 2003–4 it had 1,400 staff, with operating costs of £64.6 million (excluding the costs of sales). From April 2006 the agency will be outsourced and its services commissioned on behalf of the NHS by the Purchasing and Supply Agency (PASA).

ensure that medicines and healthcare products meet standards of safety, quality and effectiveness, and are used safely. It licenses drugs and through a system of inspection and 'post-marketing' surveillance ensures that medical devices for sale or use in the UK meet safety, quality and performance standards. It also records, monitors, and investigates reports about adverse incidents, and monitors and enforces standards of advertising, marketing, promotion and labelling. A major role assigned to the Agency is the inspection of non-commercial research clinical trials which are being undertaken in NHS trusts, for which it will recover the costs from the trusts (see Chapter 7, pages 141–2). With 747 staff in 2003–4, the Agency's operating costs were £55.8 million.[10] Its pharmaceutical activities operate as a trading fund which largely recovers its operating costs from fees and charges paid by the pharmaceutical industry. The DH is considering the extension of this principle to cover its medical devices work.

The National Programme for Information Technology (NPfIT)

The National Programme for Information Technology has been given time-limited executive agency status, for three to five years, from April 2005. Its function is to deliver an integrated information technology system across the NHS in England by 2010, with a reliable IT infrastructure linking all 18,000 NHS locations and sites through a broadband network connection known as N3. This will facilitate the development of the government's 'choose and book' initiative by making it possible for patients to book hospital appointments on-line. It will also create an electronic care records service providing each patient with an integrated electronic record of every health and social care event they experience (including all treatments received, drug allergies, etc.), and permit the electronic transmission of prescriptions from hospitals and GP surgeries to pharmacies. Other elements of the programme include a picture archiving and communications system, to make possible the display, distribution and storage of digital medical images.

The IT infrastructure resulting from the programme is also being used to facilitate financial payments. The electronic extraction and transfer of 'quality' and activity data is used in the re-imbursement of both GPs (through a system known as the 'quality management and analysis system' or QMAS) and hospital providers (through a system known as the 'secondary uses services' or SUS).

The programme is organised around five regional 'clusters' or groupings of SHAs, each of which has a local service provider responsible for providing the services. By 2004 the programme had awarded contracts worth £6.2 billion to private sector suppliers of IT services, while annual central funding was due to rise to £1.2 billion by 2005–6. By 2008 the annual costs of the programme are expected to be 4 per cent of total NHS expenditure (in the region of £3 billion).[13]

Special health authorities

Special health authorities are responsible for providing specific national services to the NHS or the public. They are established under secondary legislation and so can only carry out functions already conferred by Parliament on the Secretary of State for Health. They are thus subject to ministerial direction and accountable to the Secretary of State. As NHS bodies their work is overseen by boards with both executive and non-executive members who are collectively responsible for the services they provide. By mid-2008 there will be a total of eight special health authorities (see Table 2.2).

The NHS Institute for Learning Skills and Innovation (NHS ILSI)

This institute was established by merging the NHS Modernisation Agency with the NHS University and a proposed new innovation centre. This took place in July 2005, creating an NHS Institute for Learning Skills and Innovation to promote excellence, learning and innovation across the healthcare system in England. The Modernisation Agency and the NHS University have been dissolved, but their functions continue to be the general responsibility of the NHS ILSI (which is described further in Chapter 6, pages 124–6).

The Modernisation Agency was introduced in *The NHS Plan* and established as part of the DH in April 2001. Intended to emulate the 'change management' approach of the private sector, it worked across the whole NHS, helping clinicians and managers to spread best practice and stimulate change. Its two main roles were to modernise services, to ensure that they meet the needs and convenience of patients as outlined in the NHS Plan, and to develop current and future NHS leaders and managers. By 2003–4 it had ten teams undertaking a number of different programmes, with 765 staff and operating costs of £232 million.[10] Since its absorption into the NHS ILSI much of its work has been devolved to local NHS bodies. A smaller national modernisation team now forms part of the NHS ILSI, undertaking 'diagnostic analysis' of service problems and designing new improvement programmes.

The NHS University was established in November 2003, to support education, training and development within the NHS and form a key part of a 'lifelong learning' agenda for NHS staff. It began piloting programmes and services in November 2004, offering face-to-face as well as electronic distance-based learning, in generic subjects such as personal development toolkits and in specific subject matters such as pre-operative assessment. It operated through a network of existing educational institutions, chiefly colleges and universities. In 2003–4 it had 234 staff and operating costs of £27.8 million.[10] Core funding was provided by the DH, the costs of learning programs and services being charged to local NHS organisations and in some cases, the participants themselves. This work continues within the NHS ILSI.

The new national innovation centre incorporated within the NHS ILSI was intended to help stimulate innovation within the NHS and to facilitate the development and commercialisation of innovations coming from the NHS, academia, and the global healthcare industry. As well as co-ordinating the work of the NHS's nine regional innovation 'hubs', which offer advice and support for NHS staff who want to develop innovations, the centre should act as a 'broker' between the NHS, industry, and finance, and introduce an 'innovation fund' to help the NHS develop and exploit innovative products and procedures.

The Business Services Authority (BSA)

This authority was formed in October 2005 out of NHS Pensions Agency, the Prescription Pricing Authority, the Dental Practice Board and the NHS Counter Fraud and Security Management Service. It undertakes centralised payments and handles transactions in the work areas of these former agencies. Its services are commissioned on behalf of the NHS by the reconfigured NHS Purchasing and Supply Agency described above (pages 21–2). The easiest way to describe the BSA is to outline the work of the agencies it has absorbed:

The NHS Pensions Agency was previously an executive agency of the DH but became a special health authority in April 2004. In 2003–4 it had 277 staff and operating costs of £19 million.[10] It operated the NHS pensions scheme for both England and Wales, which has 1.99 million employed and retired members, receiving contributions totalling £3.2 billion a year and paying benefits of £3.1 billion.[11] It also operated the NHS Injury Benefit Scheme and NHS student bursaries, assessing, paying and reviewing NHS-funded healthcare students.

The Prescription Pricing Authority processed payments for supplying drugs and appliances (such as NHS wheelchairs) to pharmacists, appliance contractors and GPs. It issued Prescription Pre-Payment and other exemption certificates, (such as maternity and low-income exemptions), and produced the Drug Tariff which details the list of reimbursable items and their reimbursement prices. In 2003–4 it had 2,919 staff, with operating costs of £64.8 million.[10]

The Dental Practice Board processed payment claims to dentists, calculating and making payments to them for undertaking NHS work in England and Wales; in 2002–3 it approved remuneration of almost £1.7 billion to some 20,272 dentists. It also managed the Dental Reference Service, which provided independent dental examinations for those seeking second opinions. In 2003–4 it had 325 staff, with gross operating costs of £23.9 million.[10]

The NHS Counter Fraud and Security Management Service was established in 1998 and was responsible for developing policy and undertaking activities to prevent, detect and investigate fraud and corruption in the DH and the NHS, and to manage security. In 2003–4 it had 250 staff and operating costs of £13.3 million.[10] Only its national policy element and a core unit of 'operational expertise' have been retained within the Business Services Authority. The routine work of fraud prevention and security has been devolved to local NHS organisations.

The NHS Litigation Authority (NHSLA)

The NHS Litigation Authority was established in November 1995 to administer schemes set up by the Secretary of State for Health which enable NHS organisations to pool the cost of claims for clinical negligence and other litigation (see Table 2.3). It also handles clinical negligence claims and retains a panel of expert legal

Table 2.3   Risk-pooling schemes for clinical negligence claims administered by the NHS Litigation Authority, 2005

Name	Function
Clinical negligence scheme for trusts	Covers liabilities for alleged clinical negligence where the original incident occurred on or after 1 April 1995
Existing liabilities scheme	Covers liabilities for clinical negligence incidents which occurred before 1 April 1995
Ex Regional Health Authority scheme	Covers outstanding liabilities for clinical negligence in respect of the former Regional Health Authorities when they were abolished in April 1996
Liability to third party scheme	Covers liability to any third party where the original incident occurred on or after 1 April 1999
Property expenses scheme	Covers loss or damage to property where the original loss occurred on or after 1 April 1999

Source: Department of Health, *Departmental Report 2005*, Annex C, London.

advisers to provide advice on individual cases. In 2003–4 it had 182 staff and operating costs of £11.2 million.[10]

In 2003–4 the Authority received 3,819 claims against NHS bodies for non-clinical negligence, and 6,251 claims of clinical negligence. In the same year £423 million was paid out in connection with clinical negligence claims, including both the damages paid to patients and the legal costs borne by the NHS. Total liabilities (the theoretical cost of paying all outstanding claims immediately, including those which have occurred but have not yet been reported), were estimated at £7.78 billion for clinical claims and £100 million for non-clinical claims.[14] It is intended that the Authority will oversee the work of a scheme intended to reduce the costs of such claims, the proposed NHS Redress Scheme, described in Chapter 6 (page 135).

In April 2005 the Litigation Authority also took over the functions of a former special health authority, the Family Health Service Appeal Authority (FHSAA). The FHSAA's role was to provide rapid resolution of disputes between primary care trusts and family health services practitioners; its decisions could only be overturned by the High Court. The FHSAA's remit also encompassed disciplinary procedures for GPs and dental practitioners. Practitioners could appeal to the Appeal Authority if they were found by the Primary Care Trust (PCT) commissioning their services to be in breach of their terms of service (such as failing to undertake a consultation or provide a home visit), or if there was a dispute over their 'practice payments' – the payments GP practices receive from primary care trusts for providing primary care services – or in the case of GP registrars (GPs in training), their salaries. NHS dentists could also appeal in disputes over payments for NHS services. In addition the Authority determined appeals about entry to the 'pharmaceutical list', the list of registered practitioners whom PCTs allow to dispense drugs and medicines in their locality: pharmacists and GPs could appeal to the Authority if a PCT rejected their application to provide pharmaceutical services.

In 2003–4 the Authority had 13 staff, with operating costs of £954 million.[10] In the same year, using a panel of legal advisers, it determined 547 appeals, held 162 hearings, and carried out over 13,000 regulatory checks on practitioners.

The Health and Social Care Information Centre (HSCIC)

In April 2005 a new Health and Social Care Information Centre was formed by combining the information functions of the DH statistics division and the NHS Information Authority. Its role is to co-ordinate information requirements across the health and social care systems of England, setting data standards, carrying out the co-ordinated collection of data, analysing results and facilitating information flows.

Before the formation of the new centre the DH statistics division collected a large number of statistical returns from NHS organisations, ranging from information on the NHS workforce to information on hospital admissions and waiting times. The HSCIC took over this responsibility, although as the new market develops the scope of centrally collected and comparable statistics seems likely to narrow.

The role of the former NHS Information Authority (NHSIA) was to support the sharing and use of information throughout the NHS. This encompassed varied activities, such as procuring a new digital radio service for the Ambulance services, supporting the users of NHS data and information systems, and developing the datasets which detailed the information which NHS providers were required to collect (such as hospital activity data). In 2003–4 it had just over 900 staff and operating costs of £205 million.[10]

The National Patient Safety Agency (NPSA)

The National Patient Safety Agency was established in July 2001. Discussed more fully in Chapter 6 (page 126), it provides services to both England and Wales. Its aim is to improve the safety of NHS care, managing a national system for recording, analysing, and learning from 'adverse incidents' and 'near-misses'. It is funded by the DH, with a proportional contribution from the National Assembly for Wales. In 2003–4 it had 149 staff and operating costs of £17 million.[10]

In April 2005 the NPSA also took over the functions of the National Clinical Assessment Authority, which provided support to local NHS organisations dealing with doctors or dentists whose performance had given cause for concern. The NPSA now provides this service as a National Clinical Assessment Service, giving advice on the local handling of cases, and where necessary carrying out clinical performance assessments and making recommendations on how difficulties might be resolved (for example by remedial training). This service is provided on the basis of 'full cost recovery', NHS organisations being charged for it. In 2003–4, immediately before it was taken into the NPSA, the National Clinical Assessment Authority had 71 staff and operating costs of £6 million.[10]

The NPSA is also responsible for improving the 'patient environment', including the standards of hospital food (as part of the Better Hospital Food Programme), hospital cleanliness (which includes patient safety issues such as MRSA), and safe hospital design. In April 2005 it also became responsible for National Confidential Enquiries,[*] and assumed responsibility for supporting and overseeing the work of research ethics committees. (Research ethics committees review applications for clinical trials that involve research on patients or the public, ensuring that patient consent and other ethical issues have been considered.)

The National Institute for Health and Clinical Excellence (NICE)

The National Institute for Health and Clinical Excellence was formed in April 2005, when the National Institute for Clinical Excellence absorbed the functions of the Health Development Agency, although it is still known by its original acronym, NICE. As described in Chapter 6 (pages 113–14), its remit encompasses England and Wales, providing authoritative information for patients, the public, and healthcare professionals on evidence-based best practice in the prevention and treatment of ill-health. This remit encompasses diagnostic techniques, medicines, medical devices, the clinical management of specific conditions, and public health interventions to improve population health.

NICE was established in February 1999 to review clinical and cost-effectiveness evidence and to provide advice and guidance to NHS organisations, healthcare professionals and the public. This work falls into three broad areas: producing clinical guidelines for the management of particular conditions; publishing appraisal guidance on specific health interventions such as drugs; and publishing guidance on the safety and efficacy of interventional procedures. The work is done by independent committees, composed of healthcare professionals and people familiar with the issues affecting patients and their carers, which undertake reviews and develop guidance. In 2003–4 NICE had 81 staff and operating costs of £17.6 million.[10]

With the establishment of the new National Institute for Health and Clinical Excellence NICE's remit was extended to take on the functions of the Health Development Agency, i.e. providing guidance on best practice in the prevention of ill-health. Discussed more fully in Chapter 4 (page 75), the Health Development

---

* National Confidential Enquiries were previously the responsibility of the National Institute for Clinical Excellence. Confidential enquiries examine the events and care surrounding deaths in specific instances, to identify changes in clinical practice that will improve the quality of care and ultimately improve patients' outcomes. There are three kinds of enquiry: The National Confidential Inquiry into Suicide and Homicide (NCISH), which examines suicides and homicides by people using mental health services; The Confidential Enquiry into Maternal and Child Health (CEMACH), which examines the care of babies, children and mothers; and The National Confidential Enquiry into Patient Outcome and Death (NCEPOD), which examines cases of patients who have received a surgical or medical intervention.

Agency was established in 2000 to promote public health by gathering evidence on the effectiveness of public health interventions and providing guidance on good practice. In 2003–4 it had 132 staff and operating costs of £13 million.[10]

The National Treatment Agency for Substance Misuse (NTA)

This agency was established in April 2001 as a joint initiative in England between the DH and the Home Office. Its role is to focus efforts on drug treatment services in order to improve local treatment standards and achieve the government's main targets for reducing substance misuse by 2008. It does this by working with the Healthcare Commission (see below pages 30–1, and Chapter 6, pages 116–20) and SHAs to 'challenge' local Drug Action Teams* to improve their standards and service delivery. It does this by providing national guidance on models of care to be provided locally, setting maximum waiting times targets for access to treatment, and collecting data on the performance of services (waiting times, the number of people employed in drug treatment services, and the number of people in treatment). It also has a 'workforce strategy' to encourage professionals to work in the field of treatment for substance misuse. In 2003–4 the agency had 79 staff, with operating costs of £9.1 million.[10] In the longer term it is intended that the work of the agency will be 'main-streamed', i.e. incorporated into action at regional and local level, with SHAs leading the delivery of drug treatment services.

NHS Blood and Transplant (NHS BT)

In October 2005 a new national body known as NHS Blood and Transplant took over the functions of the former National Blood Authority and UK Transplant. Its role is to support the donation and safe use of human tissues by promoting the donation of blood and organs, coordinating a 24 hour organ-recipient matching and allocation service, and tracking the collection, preparation and distribution of blood products. However its position as a special health authority is to be reviewed, to determine whether it should be established as an independent 'public benefit corporation' – a non-profit, financially autonomous body of the kind exemplified by Foundation Trusts, described in Chapter 4, pages 63–6 and to determine whether its regulatory functions should be taken over by the new Regulatory Authority for Fertility and Tissue (see below, pages 33–4).

The National Blood Authority was responsible for the management of the National Blood Service in England and Wales, collecting blood from voluntary donors, processing it and supplying it to hospitals.[11] In 2002–3 it collected over 2 million units of blood and supplied over 300 hospitals. It also encompassed the work of the International Blood Group Reference Laboratory, which provides a reference service and issues diagnostic material, and the Bio Products Laboratory,

---

* Drug Action Teams (DATs) are local networks drawing together the key agencies involved with substance misuse, such as health, the police and probation services, and drug treatment services.

which makes therapeutic products from blood plasma. In 2003–4 it had almost 6,000 staff and operating costs of £365 million,[10] costs which were largely recouped through charges to hospitals for blood handling, and through the sale of bio products.

UK Transplant (UKT) was formed from a predecessor authority in July 2000. It co-ordinated organ donation throughout the UK and Republic of Ireland, in order to maximise the availability and equitable distribution of organs. It held the NHS organ donor register, and was responsible for publicity and national campaigns. In 2003–4 it had 121 staff and operating costs of £10.5 million.[10] It was funded by the DH, with Scotland, Wales and Northern Ireland contributing agreed proportions.

Executive non-departmental public bodies

NHS executive non-departmental public bodies are independent bodies which perform specific national functions on behalf of the NHS or the public. Unlike special health authorities, however, they are set up under primary legislation, which gives them powers independent of the Secretary of State for Health. Their work is overseen by boards made up of both executive and non-executive members, who are collectively responsible for the services provided. They operate to a greater or lesser extent at arm's length from ministers, being directly accountable to Parliament.

By April 2008 there will be eight executive non-departmental public bodies providing services to the NHS (see Table 2.2), the first two – Monitor and the Healthcare Commmission – being the most important:

Monitor (the independent regulator of NHS foundation trusts)

Monitor was established in April 2004 under legislation provided in the 2003 Health and Social Care (Community Health and Standards) Act. Described more fully in Chapter 6 (pages 112–13), its role is to grant licences to operate to NHS foundation trusts, and then to monitor their observance of the terms of the licences. In 2003–4 it had 28 staff and operating costs of £2.8 million.[10] As an executive non-departmental public body it has its own statutory powers, including power to regulate its own procedures. Its board members are, however, appointed by the Secretary of State for Health, and it is accountable through her or him to Parliament, submitting annual reports on how it has exercised its powers and functions. Its status as a non-departmental public body is, however, to be reviewed. Subject to legislation it may be established as a non-ministerial government department, accountable directly to Parliament.

The Healthcare Commission

The Healthcare Commission, whose full name is the Commission for Healthcare Audit and Inspection (CHAI), was established in April 2004 under the 2003

Health and Social Care (Community Health and Standards Act). Its functions are described more fully in Chapter 6 (page 116–17); its singular role is to inspect all healthcare services in England, including non-NHS services. It publishes its findings, as well as reporting directly to Parliament. The Commission also has a limited role in Wales, reporting to the Welsh Assembly on the state of NHS services in Wales (see Chapter 9, page 168).

For NHS organisations the Commission inspects services, publishes annual performance ratings, and recommends remedial action where required. It undertakes NHS 'value for money' studies, scrutinises patient complaints, and investigates serious failures in NHS services, such as allegations of abuse or higher-than-expected mortality figures. The Commission also inspects and licenses independent healthcare services, and inspects foundation trusts – for the latter reporting its findings to the independent regulator, Monitor. The Healthcare Commission is currently funded by the DH, but the DH intends that for independent (non-NHS) healthcare providers the Commission will move toward 'full cost recovery', charging for the full cost of its inspections.

The Healthcare Commission has its head office in London and regional offices in Bristol, Leeds, Manchester and Nottingham. It is 'led' by a board of 14 Commissioners drawn from healthcare professionals, such as a professor of cardiac surgery and a physician for the elderly, as well as from people working for charities and health policy think-tanks. It has a senior management team of seven, and uses over 1,000 'reviewers' to undertake its inspections, drawn from the full range of healthcare professions. It has about 600 support staff. Its budget for 2005–6 was £78.7 million.[15]

On its formation in 2004 the Commission subsumed the work of the Commission for Health Inspection (CHI), the National Care Standards Commission, and the 'value for money' work of the Audit Commission. However its remit is to be further extended by taking over the functions of Mental Health Act Commission to regulate care for people detained under the Mental Health Act. By 2008 it is also to merge with the Commission for Social Care Inspection (CSCI), its counterpart for the inspection of social care. Itself established in April 2004, the Commission for Social Care Inspection inspects and licenses public, private and voluntary social care services, such as nursing and residential care homes and domiciliary services, for both adults and children. It also publishes performance ratings and reports directly to Parliament. The merging of the two organisations will result in a single body responsible for the inspection of all health and social care services.

The NHS Appointments Commission

The NHS Appointments Commission was established in April 2001 to meet the commitment in *The NHS Plan* that NHS organisations should have the highest quality non-executive leadership. Initially a special health authority, it will be re-established as an executive non-departmental public body from April 2006, allowing it to take on functions additional to those that can be delegated by the Secretary of State for Health.

It comprises a chair and eight regional commissioners (themselves experienced non-executive members of NHS organisations), each of whom is responsible for the integrity of the appointments process in his or her region. The Commission is responsible for appointing chairs and non-executive members to the boards of health authorities, NHS trusts and Primary Care Trusts, and now also makes the majority of non-executive appointments to national 'arms-length bodies' (executive agencies, special health authorities, and non-departmental public bodies such as the Healthcare Commission). With a total of some 4,000 chairs and non-executive members on NHS boards, appointed for three to five years, up to 1,500 appointments are made annually.[16] The Commission is also responsible for appointing members to patient and public involvement forums, and for the regular appraisal of their chairs and members (see Chapter 6, pages 129–30), and for appointing lay members to hospital research ethics committees. NHS foundation trusts can also pay the Commission to recruit their non-executive or 'lay' board members, and under forthcoming legislation the Commission may also be granted power to make appointments to non-NHS organisations too.

The Commission is responsible for ensuring that the appointments process is open and transparent. It follows a code of practice laid down by the Office of the Commissioner for Public Appointments, appointing candidates on criteria determined by the Secretary of State for Health. Appointment panels for chairs consist of one or more regional commissioners and an independent assessor, while for non-executive members they consist of chairs from two local NHS organisations and an independent assessor. Trained and accredited by the Appointments Commission, in conjunction with the Office of Commissioner for Public Appointments, their role is to ensure that the guidelines laid down by the Commissioner for Public Appointments are followed in a fair and consistent manner.

The Commission is also responsible for ensuring that chairs and non-executive board members receive proper induction and training, and that they are appraised on an annual basis: a national appraisal process was established in March 2002. This is based on a review of their performance against objectives set prospectively by the individuals in question, in conjunction with the assessor; for chairs the objectives include the performance of the organisation itself.

The Commission is accountable to the DH for managing its budget, but is held to account by the Commissioner for Public Appointments for the quality of its work. The Commission is required to provide her office with annual statistical returns, and has its processes and working practices inspected annually by her auditors. In 2003–4 the NHS Appointments Commission had 46 staff and operating costs of £4.3 million.[10]

The Council for the Regulation of Healthcare Professionals

Also known as the Council for Healthcare Regulatory Excellence, this Council was established in 2003. Described in more detail in Chapter 6 (page 122), its role is to oversee the nine regulatory bodies for healthcare professionals.* Serving the interests of patients and the public, it determines the principles of good regulation and ensures that regulators conform to them in a consistent manner. In 2003–4, its first year of operation, it had three staff and operating costs of £1.4 million.[10]

The Health Protection Agency (HPA)

The Health Protection Agency was established in England and Wales in April 2003. Initially a special health authority, it subsequently became a UK-wide non-departmental public body, enabling it to perform functions beyond those that can be delegated by the Secretary of State for Health. Discussed more fully in Chapter 4 (pages 75–7) it is responsible for health protection functions relating to biological, chemical and radiological hazards, and emergency planning. It has subsumed the work of the Public Health Laboratory Service; the National Poisons Information Centre; the National Focus for Chemical Incidents (and its regional service provider units, which support the management of chemical incidents); and the work of Consultants in Communicable Disease Control, and regional emergency planning advisers. In 2005 it also took over the work of the former National Radiological Protection Board,† and by April 2006 will take over the functions of the National Institute for Biological Standards and Control, which standardises and controls the biological materials used in medicines. In 2003–4 the HPA had over 2,500 staff and operating costs of £172.5 million.[10]

The Regulatory Authority for Fertility and Tissue (RAFT)

By April 2008 a new body is to be established, the Regulatory Authority for Fertility and Tissue, or RAFT, which will combine the work of the Human Fertilisation and Embryology Authority and the Human Tissue Authority. As a UK-wide body it will set standards and enforce compliance, covering all aspects of the use of embryos and human tissues in both research and therapy. This will encompass some areas outside health care, such as sperm-banks and university medical and anatomy schools.

Meantime its two predecessor bodies continue to function. The Human Fertilisation and Embryology Authority (HFEA) was established in 1991 to regulate human fertility work. It licenses and monitors clinics undertaking IVF and donor insemination, licenses research involving the use or creation of embryos

---

*   The General Medical Council, the General Dental Council, the General Optical Council, the Nursing and Midwifery Council, the Health Professions Council, the General Chiropractic Council, the General Osteopathic Council, the Royal Pharmaceutical Society of Great Britain, and the Pharmaceutical Society of Northern Ireland.

†   Established in 1970, the NRPB conducted research into and provided advice on the effects and health risks of radiation, radiation measurement and dose assessment, the environmental impact of nuclear discharges and waste disposal, emergency planning and nuclear accidents.

in vitro, and regulates the storage of gametes and embryos. In 2003–4 it had 106 staff and operating costs of £7.3 million.[10]

The Human Tissue Authority (HTA) is an interim body, established with a 'shadow' board in April 2005 and intended to be fully functioning by April 2006. It is intended to address concerns regarding the storage and use of human tissue within medical and academic settings such as medical schools, following the high-profile investigation into the retention of human tissue at Alder Hey hospital in Liverpool in 2001. It will develop standards and codes of practice, and implement operational and inspection procedures.

The Postgraduate Medical Education and Training Board (PMETB)

This board was established in April 2003, but became fully operational in September 2005. It has UK-wide responsibility for overseeing postgraduate medical and dental education. This includes developing and approving programmes of postgraduate training, setting entry standards and approving curricula, and recruiting, developing and assessing educational supervisors. It also sets the standards for the certificate of completion of training for both general practitioners and hospital specialists, issues the certificates, and recommends entry (i.e. admission) to the General Medical Council's register of accredited practitioners and hospital consultants (the 'specialist register').

The Board has 19 medical and six lay members. The Secretary of State for Health appoints 19 members, and the devolved administrations in Scotland, Wales and Northern Ireland appoint one medical and one lay member each. In its first year of operation (2003–4) the Board's operating costs were £3 million.[10]

The General Social Care Council

The General Social Care Council acts on behalf of the DH to register individual social care workers, such as those working in care homes and providing domiciliary services. It also regulates their training and professional conduct. In 2003–4 it had 146 staff and operating costs of almost £10 million.[10]

Other bodies: tribunals and judicial authorities

A number of non-departmental tribunals or independent judicial authorities exist to review and determine appeals relating to the DH or the NHS. Mental Health Review Tribunals review applications or references relating to the compulsory detention of patients under the Mental Health Act. In 2002–3 they held 10,076 hearings on 21,202 applications. Secretariat support was provided by 73 DH staff, with administrative costs of £2.4 million.[11] A new Family Health Services Appeal Authority, formed in December 2001,* deals with appeals made by providers of

---

*   Not to be confused with the old FHSAA (special health authority) referred to above on pages 26–7, which was absorbed into the Litigation Authority. The new FHSAA is not a

primary care in England and Wales. These are appeals against decisions such as the suspension or removal of a practitioner from a PCT's list of registered providers, or the refusal of an application to join a list. Between June 2004 and July 2005 it heard 43 appeals, with secretariat services provided by the Litigation Authority.[17] The Pharmaceutical Price Control Tribunal determines appeals from suppliers and manufacturers of NHS medicines against decisions made by the Secretary of State for Health, such as decisions limiting prices or profits or refusing approval for a price increase. Its staff consists of one clerk; at the time of writing there had been no appeals to this tribunal. The independent judicial nature of all these bodies is indicated by the fact that their members are appointed by the Lord Chancellor, not the Secretary of State for Health.

special health authority but an independent tribunal and deals with a somewhat different range of issues from those of the former FHSAA (special health authority).

3 Organisations commissioning services

Organisations commissioning or 'purchasing' healthcare services on behalf of patients hold a central position within the NHS. This function is currently performed on behalf of geographically defined populations by organisations known as Primary Care Trusts. A number of other commissioning bodies are, however, also being developed. These include GP practices commissioning services for the general population, as well as bodies commissioning services for vulnerable populations, such as care trusts commissioning services for the elderly and people with mental health problems, and children's trusts commissioning services for children.

Primary Care Trusts

Establishment

Since April 2002 Primary Care Trusts or PCTs have been responsible for commissioning primary, secondary, and community healthcare services for their local populations. PCTs were first introduced in the 1997 white paper *The New NHS. Modern, Dependable,* replacing Primary Care Groups (PCGs) – geographically defined groups of general practices covering average populations of about 100,000. The entire population of England is now covered by 303 PCTs, with average populations of 170,000, although they vary considerably in size (see Table 3.1). Almost 90 per cent of them have boundaries co-terminous with those of local authorities.[1]

Since their establishment a number of PCTs have, in fact, merged in all but name, being organised into 'clusters' with joint management teams, to make better use of scarce managerial and organisational capacity. PCT 'networks' have also been mentioned;[2] although poorly described at the time of writing, these networks are presumably groups of PCTs similar to the existing 'clusters' just mentioned. The DH has, however, indicated its intention of reducing the number of PCTs to less than 100, to make them larger organisations covering larger populations (of around 500,000). These new PCTs should in principle have boundaries aligned with those of local authority social services departments. The reconfiguration of

Table 3.1 Primary Care Trusts in England by
population range, as established in April 2002

Population range	Number of PCTs
0–99,999	38
100,000–149,999	104
150,000–199,999	77
200,000–249,999	44
250,000–299,999	26
300,000+	14
Total	303

Source: Department of Health, personal communication.

PCTs is to be overseen by SHAs; the DH intends that the changes be completed
by October 2006.

Function

The role of PCTs is to improve the health of the community, to secure high
quality primary, secondary and community care services, and to integrate local
health and social care services (see Table 3.2). This makes them responsible for
commissioning, or overseeing the commissioning by GP practices (see pages
43–4), of the full range of healthcare and community services for their local
populations. For this purpose the PCTs now receive over 80 per cent of the total
NHS budget.[3]

The planning function

As the lead planners for the NHS at the local level PCTs are responsible for
identifying the healthcare needs of their local populations and incorporating them
into annual Local Delivery Plans. These plans should describe planned health and
service improvements in each PCT's area over the next three years, and are also
considered an important tool in the drive to develop alternatives to hospital care,
reducing inappropriate hospital admissions, and helping to develop services in
'accessible high-street locations'.[4] PCTs undertake the planning of services in the
context of a national 'planning framework' which sets out national priority areas
and their related targets for a three-year period. For the period 2005–6 to 2007–8 the
framework covered four national priority areas drawn from the DH's public service
agreements with the Treasury:* the health and well-being of the population, long-
term medical conditions, access to services, and patients' and users' experience.

---

* As described in Chapter 6 (page 109), the DH is accountable to the Treasury through
  public service agreements which set out measurable targets for the work of the DH,
  such as reducing mortality from cancer.

Table 3.2   Roles and responsibilities of Primary Care Trusts

Role	Responsibility
Improving the health of the community	Leading on public health issues Developing three-year local delivery plans Engaging in partnership work and community-based health and care initiatives
Planning and securing the provision of services	Implementing population screening programmes Administering, developing and integrating family health services, medical (primary care), dental and optical Securing all mental health, emergency ambulance and patient transport services, NHS Direct and walk-in centres Overseeing the commissioning of community and secondary care services* Commissioning tertiary/specialised services
Integrating health and social care	Working with local authorities, social services, and voluntary organisations

Source: Adapted from Department of Health, *Shifting the Balance of Power, Securing Delivery*, 2001, London.

Note
* With the introduction of GP practice-based commissioning PCTs will be responsible only for commissioning specialised services – they will oversee the commissioning of secondary and community health care services by GP practices.

These priority areas contained 20 national targets for PCTs to achieve, working in conjunction with service providers (see Chapter 6, pages 109–10).[5]

Partnerships with local authorities

PCTs also take the lead in partnership work with local authorities and other agencies in order to improve health and promote health education, community development and social and economic regeneration. The 1999 Health Act enabled them to pool resources with local authorities so that they can undertake joint commissioning or 'purchasing' of social care services for groups requiring both health and social care services, such as the elderly and those with mental health problems.

Primary and community care services

PCTs secure primary care services through contracts with GP practices.* Since December 2004 they have also been responsible for securing the provision of

* GPs' services have traditionally been provided by independent general practitioners, through a nationally-agreed contract framework known as General Medical Services (GMS). Since 1998 locally developed contracts known as Personal Medical Services (PMS) have also been introduced, so as to be more responsive to local needs (for example in deprived or under-doctored areas) by employing staff in a greater variety of ways, including GPs on salary.

'out-of-hours' GP services; in some instances these are still provided by individual GP practices, but they are increasingly provided by GP 'co-operatives'. This encompasses a variety of working arrangements, such as groups of practices providing joint out-of-hours cover for their patients, or individual GPs undertaking extra shifts on behalf of a centrally-run co-operative. Since April 2004 PCTs have also been able to purchase 'specialised' primary care services (such as out-of-hours services) from 'alternative providers'.* These may be either commercial or 'not for profit' healthcare organisations, other PCTs, or even NHS hospital trusts or foundation trusts.

PCTs also oversee the provision of services by other family health service providers such as pharmacists and optometrists, and since April 2005, NHS dentistry services. They are also responsible for ensuring the provision of community health services, such as district nursing, health visiting, family planning, chiropody, physiotherapy and rehabilitation services. They 'secure' these services either by commissioning ('purchasing') them from other providers, or by directly providing them themselves. The DH publication *Commissioning a Patient-Led NHS*, however, laid out the DH's intention that by December 2008 PCTs should provide such services only where it is not possible to commission them from a separate provider.

These community health services are provided through GP practices, community health centres and community hospitals as well as in people's own homes. There is an increasing emphasis on the use of such services to provide care closer to home for patients with chronic conditions, both to improve patients' experience and to help avoid hospital admissions. One way PCTs are achieving this is through new arrangements which allow PCTs to provide them directly by employing their own staff, under arrangements known as PCT medical services (PCT MS). For example the Castle Point and Rochford PCT employs nurses with a special interest in diabetes. They run nurse-led community clinics and drop-in clinics which effectively function as an 'out-reach' service. By 2005 nine PCTs were also implementing and evaluating a nurse-led chronic disease management programme for vulnerable elderly patients known as the 'Evercare' project, through a high-profile collaboration with an American corporation called United Healthcare.† The previously mentioned intention of the DH that PCTs cease to provide community health services makes the continuation and/or development of such schemes unlikely.

---

* New contracting arrangements known as Alternative Provider Medical Services (APMS) were introduced in the 2003 Health and Social Care (Community Health and Standards) Act. They were expected to be used mainly for the provision of specialised services (such as out-of-hours services), but can also be used for the provision of general medical (primary care) services.

† This involves providing case-management to oversee and co-ordinate the provision of services for vulnerable elderly people. The DH intends that this approach should be disseminated throughout the NHS and adopted by every PCT between 2005 and 2008, with over 3,000 community matrons providing case management services for 250,000 patients with complex needs.

Thirty-one PCTs also have teaching status, with the aim of attracting high-calibre staff to work in deprived areas. They offer clinical posts to GPs and other healthcare professionals, with an emphasis on learning, research and development.

Secondary care services

PCTs commission secondary care services from secondary care providers. In the past these have been NHS trusts (a generic term encompassing acute hospital trusts, specialist trusts providing specific services such as orthopaedics or learning disability services, mental health trusts[7], and ambulance trusts). Commissioning secondary care from these providers involves NHS contracts or 'service level agreements', which are not legally binding but which are overseen by the Secretary of State for Health.

More recently PCTs have also begun to commission services from newly-established NHS foundation trusts, and from hospitals in the 'independent' (private and voluntary) sector. This commissioning involves legally binding contracts. PCTs are also able to commission some elective services, such as diagnostic and surgical procedures, from both NHS and 'Independent Sector Treatment Centres' or ISTCs (described in Chapter 4, pages 66–7). The intention is that from 2006 onwards PCTs should be commissioning secondary care services in such a way that patients can choose from at least four or five different providers of elective care (i.e. planned, non-emergency treatment, such as hip replacements and cataracts). From 2008 onwards patients should be able to choose from any provider – NHS, private, or voluntary – that meets NHS standards of care and is willing to be paid at the rates set in the national 'tariff' (see Chapter 5, pages 97–8).

The introduction of GP practice-based commissioning in April 2005 is described below (see pages 43–4). With this, the commissioning role of PCTs is set to alter. GP practices are increasingly taking responsibility for commissioning services, determining the type and level of services to be purchased and which provider they are to be purchased from. PCTs will be responsible only for ensuring that the commissioning decisions of GP practices conform to national and local objectives and targets. PCTs will also assume an 'agency' role, ensuring that practices stay within their budgets; making the contracts with providers on behalf of practices; and monitoring the activity undertaken within the contracts.

Specialist services

PCTs are also responsible for commissioning specialised or so called 'tertiary' services, such as cancer, neurosurgery and haemophilia services. Such services are provided in a relatively small number of specialist centres, for populations of more than a million people.[6] This work is undertaken by collaborative commissioning groups of PCTs, which may cover up to five Strategic Health Authority areas. They are responsible for planning, commissioning and funding such services, which are then overseen by one of the SHAs on behalf of the group. From April 2006 onwards PCTs will also be responsible for commissioning prison health services (85 PCTs have one or more prisons in their areas)[7], to provide prisoners with access to the same range and quality of healthcare services as the general public, and to facilitate their re-entry into mainstream health services after leaving prison.

Ongoing changes

Ongoing reform of the NHS means that the functions of PCTs are likely to remain in evolution at least for the near future. In June 2004 the DH stated that their development is to achieve 'higher priority' in the 'next stages of reform'.[8] This included PCTs 'realis[ing] the potential of commissioning', in effect using their position as the funders of services to influence the direction of local service development.

The DH also intends that all NHS organisations should eventually achieve foundation status, which will presumably include PCTs. Under the 2001 Health and Social Care Act, however, PCTs are already able to form joint ventures with organisations from the independent (private and voluntary) sector. They may undertake capital development projects through the Local Improvement Finance Trust initiative (described in Chapter 5, pages 94–5), and form joint venture companies with private companies to generate income. Such companies can be established to exploit intellectual property rights, for example selling the findings of research studies or advances in medical technology, or to provide services such as NHS-supported nursing-home accommodation.

At the same time as PCTs are to be 'developed', a number of policy initiatives will actually reduce their remit and limit their functions. The long-established policy aim of increased collaboration between PCTs and local authority social services has led to the introduction of 'care trusts' (see below, pages 44–6). This has led to some PCTs delegating their responsibility for older people's services to local care trusts. Similarly, children's trusts have recently been introduced (see below, pages 46–7), to which PCTs can delegate responsibility for commissioning and providing children's health services. Perhaps more fundamentally, as we have already noted, the development of GP practice-based commissioning will reduce if not remove PCTs' responsibility for making decisions regarding the provision and commissioning of the full range of healthcare services. PCTs will be left increasingly with an 'agency role', holding the contracts with providers, and presumably enforcing the contracts.

Structure

PCTs are established in law as independent organisations. Like other NHS organisations they are corporate bodies, whose work is overseen by boards with executive and non-executive members. Each PCT also has a 'professional executive committee' or PEC, which provides advice on clinical matters and is intended to draw local clinical expertise into the leadership of the PCT. Below these two bodies the senior management team is responsible for overseeing the day-to-day running of the PCT. Unlike other NHS organisations there is no cap on the amount of their finances that PCTs can spend on management costs. Latest figures (2002–3) put these at a total of £723 million for England,[9] or an average of £2.4 million per

PCT. The reconfiguration of PCTs described on pages 36–7 is, however, intended to deliver a reduction in management and administrative costs.

The board

The board of each PCT oversees its work and strategic direction, and is responsible for ensuring that it meets its financial, statutory, and legal responsibilities. These include the utilisation of funds, the quality of care provided, and governance arrangements.

Board membership is limited to 15 people, who must include at least five executive members of the PCT, including the chief executive, the finance director and the director of public health, plus two other members of the PEC, representing healthcare professionals and staff. The board must have a lay chair, and at least five non-executive members, enough to ensure a lay majority.[10] These non-executive members are intended to ensure that the direction of the PCT is 'in line with the local community'. They are drawn from members of the public – i.e. not NHS or civil service staff – who live in the area served by the PCT, or who are registered as patients of GPs in that area. They are self-nominated, but are selected through a process of open competition by the NHS Appointments Commission (see Chapter 2, pages 31–2).

The board must also contain a member of the patient and public involvement forum, to represent the views of patients served by the PCT (see Chapter 6, pages 129–30). One board member, usually a medical or nursing representative, is responsible for clinical governance issues, to ensure that procedures are in place to monitor and improve the quality of services provided (see Chapter 6, pages 114–16).

The professional executive committee

Each PCT has a professional executive committee or PEC which operates alongside the board. Its role is to draw local clinical expertise into the leadership of the PCT, by providing advice to the board and the senior management team on clinical matters such as priorities for service development, policy development and investment plans.

Membership of the PEC is limited to 18, and must include the chief executive, the director of finance, a senior public health professional (such as a consultant in public health, or a non-medical equivalent, being a specialist in public health), and a social services representative nominated by the local authority. The remaining members are drawn from healthcare professionals working for the PCT (GPs, dentists, nurses, pharmacists, and allied health professionals*); they must include at least one GP and one nurse, but as a group they should reflect the functions of

---

*   The 'professions allied to medicine' (PAMS) include chiropodists/podiatrists, dieticians, occupational therapists, orthoptists, physiotherapists, speech and language therapists, paramedics, radiographers, prosthetists, and drama, art and music therapists.

the PCT with no one profession in the majority. Candidates nominate themselves but are elected by their respective professional constituencies within the PCT.

The senior management team

The senior management team works with the chief executive to oversee the day-to-day running of the PCT, and is responsible for ensuring that the decisions of the board and the PEC are implemented. The team must include the director of finance, the director of public health and a senior nurse, and have a nominated lead for clinical governance issues (see Chapter 6, pages 114–16). The composition of the remainder of the team is determined by the chief executive, in discussion with the board; it varies from area to area, but typically also includes directors responsible for clinical services, clinical governance and quality issues, service development and modernisation, and corporate and human resource issues.

GP practice-based commissioning

In June 2004 the DH outlined its intention to devolve responsibility for commissioning services to GP practices. This is intended to provide an incentive for GPs to manage referrals to secondary care more effectively, leading to savings for the NHS.[11] Various models were to be established and evaluated, ranging from 'indicative budgets' (where practices are told the amount of money available, but the PCT continues to actually hold the budget) to fully devolved practice budgets.

Indicative budgets were introduced as a first step in April 2005; practices wishing to participate must agree with their PCT the specific services they wish to commission, for both planned (elective) and emergency care. The DH publication *Commissioning a Patient-led NHS* subsequently laid out the DH's intention that by December 2006 the commissioning of all community and secondary health services will be undertaken by GP practices (so-called GP practice-based commissioning), rather than by PCTs. In effect GP practices are told the budget they have available for services for the coming year. They are responsible for determining the healthcare needs of their registered patients and how these should be met, within the context of the national and local targets in the PCT's Local Delivery Plan. This means that practices must determine the type and level of services to be provided, and which providers these should be purchased from. Practices can use any savings they make for improved patient services.

The DH expects that there will be a variety of forms of commissioning groups, depending on the size of individual practices and the levels of activity for different services. Some services will be commissioned by individual practices, while other practices may choose to work in groups (known as 'localities') to commission all or some of their services. These localities are seen as a way to improve efficiency, provide larger risk-pools, and exercise a stronger influence on service re-design.

Within GP practice-based commissioning PCTs are responsible for ensuring that the commissioning decisions of practices are in line with national and local requirements, such as providing patients with a choice of hospital provider, and with the achievement of the targets in the Local Delivery Plan. PCTs also act as the 'agents' of GP commissioner practices, being responsible for determining their budgets, holding the actual funds, ensuring that practices remain within their budgets, making the contracts with providers, and monitoring the levels of activity within these contracts. PCTs are responsible for meeting any overspend by GP practices, although practices are expected to achieve financial balance over a three-year cycle by managing the way in which they refer patients for treatment. PCTs, groups of PCTs, or groups of practices may also choose to hold back a percentage of practice budgets to form a 'contingency fund', in order to meet any higher-than-expected costs due to unforeseen circumstances, such as changes in a practice's list size.

For 2005–6 GP practice budgets were set on the basis of past activity levels, i.e. on the basis of previous years' referral data. From 2006–7, however, a 'fair shares' approach will be introduced; practices will be moved towards a system where budgets are allocated on the basis of a weighted capitation formula. As described in Chapter 5 (pages 83–5), such formulae attempt to distribute resources on the basis of population (list sizes), adjusted for measures of healthcare need.

Care trusts

Establishment

Care trusts were announced in *The NHS Plan* and subsequently legislated for in the 2001 Health and Social Care Act. Intended to facilitate the delivery of integrated health and social care services, they build on flexibilities introduced by the 1999 Health Act that authorised the joint funding of health and social care services by the NHS and local authorities for groups such as older people. Thus care trusts are voluntary partnerships between NHS bodies (PCTs or NHS trusts) and the social services departments of local authorities.

As voluntary partnerships, care trusts are formed on joint application by both partners to the Secretary of State for Health, and can be dissolved on the application of either partner. The Secretary of State also has the power to impose the creation of a care trust where local health and social care organisations are deemed to be failing to establish effective partnerships, or where their services are failing.

Although care trusts are an important policy aim of the DH, by May 2005 only eight had been established, all the result of voluntary applications. The poor uptake of care trusts probably reflects their introduction during a period of ongoing reform and organisational change, with NHS organisations, and particularly PCTs, focussing on developing their own organisations. It may also reflect the very barriers between organisations which they are intended to overcome, with different organisational cultures, different ways of working and different sources of funding acting as deterrents to their establishment. Furthermore, in view of the DH's wish that PCTs should cease to provide services themselves (see page 39), their future role looks unclear.

Function

Care trusts were introduced to facilitate the delivery of integrated and co-ordinated health and social care services across organisational boundaries. They are particularly aimed at vulnerable populations with complex needs, such as the elderly and those with mental health or learning disability problems. Of the eight established by May 2005, five provide mental health services, two provide services for older people, and one, formed by a PCT, provides adult social services as well as primary and secondary healthcare services.

The way care trusts function to achieve their remit depends on their constituent organisations. Those formed by partnerships between PCTs and local authority services both commission services on behalf of their populations, and provide services to them directly. They may be responsible for the whole remit of the PCT, as well as for specific social care services. For example Northumberland Care Trust provides both primary and community care services to its population of 317,000,[12] commissions secondary care services on their behalf, and provides social care services for adults and older people with physical or learning disabilities. It also manages other social services, such as day care and home care services and residential homes, on behalf of Northumberland County Council. Alternatively PCTs can delegate specific services, such as older people's services, to a care trust. Other models include a care trust formed by a PCT which also commissions services on behalf of other PCTs.

Care trusts established by partnerships between an NHS trust (such as a mental health trust) and local authority social services have a provider function; they provide or 'sell' their services to local PCTs, GP practices and local authorities, who purchase them on behalf of the local population. Thus these care trusts can provide services to the populations of one or more PCTs and their respective local authorities, although they do not necessarily provide health and social care services to the same geographical populations. For example Bradford District Care Trust is a partnership between a community mental health trust and local authority mental health and learning disability services. Its services are commissioned by both local PCTs and the local authority on behalf of over 550,000 people.[13] It provides mental health services to the populations of five PCTs, but only provides learning disability services to four of them, learning-disabled people in the fifth being served by another local authority.

Structure

Care trusts are statutory NHS bodies, with local authority functions 'added on'. There is, however, no single model for a care trust. Both their structure and their size depend on the constituent organisations which formed them. Thus they may be formed by a PCT, to perform certain delegated functions of a PCT such as providing older people's services, or by an NHS trust such as a mental health trust. They may exercise local authority functions delegated by one or more local authority.

Like PCTs and other NHS organisations, care trusts are corporate bodies, each having a board which oversees its work and strategic direction. The board is responsible for ensuring that the care trust meets its financial, statutory, and legal responsibilities, overseeing the utilisation of funds, the quality of care provided, and governance arrangements. Board membership is similar to that of PCTs, as discussed on page 42. At least one board member, however, should be someone like a manager of local authority services, to represent the local authority's delegated functions. The executive members of the board should also reflect the function of the trust. For care trusts formed by an NHS trust (such as a mental health trust) they must include the chief executive, the director of finance, the director of nursing and a medical director. For care trusts formed by PCTs they must include the chief executive, the director of finance, the director of public health, and three members of the PEC to represent staff and professionals.

Care trusts formed by PCTs also have a professional executive committee or PEC to provide advice to the board and senior management team on clinical matters and draw clinicians into its leadership. The PEC's membership is similar to that of a PCT, as described on pages 42–3. It is limited to a maximum of 18 and should represent the functions of the care trust, with no one profession in the majority. It should also have at least one but no more than two members nominated by the local authority to represent its delegated functions.

Like PCTs, care trusts also have senior management teams to oversee the day-to-day running of the trust. Other than a mandatory requirement for the team to include the director of finance its composition depends on the functions of the care trust. It usually contains directors responsible for service delivery, the quality of services and clinical governance arrangements (see Chapter 6, pages 114–16), and corporate and human resource issues.

Children's trusts

Establishment

Children's trusts (ChTs) were introduced in the 2003 green paper *Every Child Matters*. The 2004 Children's Act subsequently provided the necessary powers, imposing a duty to co-operate on bodies involved with the well-being of children, and enabling them to pool their budgets. This was a response to a number of failings in child protection services and recommendations by enquiries, including the high-profile enquiry into the death of Victoria Climbié (a nine-year-old child who had multiple admissions to hospital that were later recognised to be due to abuse, and who was under the care of a social worker when she died).

The intention is that every local authority should have a ChT by 2008. In July 2003, 35 'pathfinder' ChTs were established in a variety of locations throughout England, to run until 2006. Their experiences and outcomes will be evaluated and used as the basis for determining the eventual model, or models, for ChTs.

Function

Children's trusts are intended to integrate local education, social services, and healthcare services for children and young people (up to age nineteen). Intended to facilitate 'joined-up working' between agencies, their principal function is one of co-ordination. ChTs provide a single organisation responsible for identifying children's needs, and a single organisation responsible for commissioning the required health, social, and education services, using pooled budgets. A ChT can also provide services itself, for example through personal advisers and key-workers attached to the ChT.

ChTs are also intended to facilitate the co-ordinated working of multi-disciplinary teams using common training material and assessment frameworks to ensure that consistent messages are conveyed. In addition they are intended to facilitate the sharing of information across organisational boundaries so that warning signs relating to vulnerable children can be aggregated and acted on.

ChTs were initially concerned primarily with vulnerable children (such as 'looked after children' – i.e. those under the care of local services) and those with specific health, social care or educational needs, but the intention is that they will eventually play a broader role in improving the well-being of all children within an area, for example by taking the lead in securing improvements in preventative health measures and on social care issues.

Structure

Children's trusts are voluntary partnerships between the health service, social services and local education services, the PCT delegating to them its responsibility for children's health services (such as community paediatrics, teenage pregnancy services and child and adolescent mental health services). Depending on the local situation a ChT can also cover children's services such as youth offending teams* and 'Sure Start' programmes.† ChTs work in partnership with other organisations involved with children, such as housing, leisure services and the police, and voluntary and community organisations such as churches.

Unlike care trusts ChTs are not separate legal entities, but are part of and led by local authorities, which have statutory duties towards children. Their responsibility for health services is delegated to them by PCTs under the 1999 Health Act, which enables PCTs to delegate functions to, and pool budgets with, local authorities. There are no requirements for their structure and governance arrangements; different models will be compared in light of the experience of the first 'pathfinder' ChTs. They will, however, be overseen by local authorities' directors of children's services, who are responsible (and accountable) for the services ChTs deliver.

---

* Multi-disciplinary teams working with young people and their families to prevent re-offending.
† These provide early years support for young people and their families, such as supported nursery places and linking parents of young children into various health and other initiatives.

4 Organisations providing services

Organisations providing NHS services are most simply categorised into those providing services outside the hospital setting (i.e. primary care services such as general practice), and 'acute' hospitals, which provide specialist, secondary care services. Some hospitals also provide tertiary care – highly specialised services such as neuro-surgery and thoracic surgery and the treatment of haemophilia. Historically hospitals have accounted for over 50 per cent of the NHS budget for service provision,[1] even though they account for only 19 per cent of the daily contacts people have with the NHS (Figure 4.1).[2] A key feature of the 'new' NHS is the drive to provide alternatives to existing hospital services, with a greater variety of service providers in both secondary and primary care, and alternatives to the provision of secondary care in the traditional hospital setting.

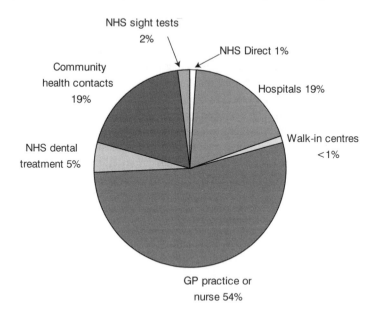

Figure 4.1　Shares of total contacts with the NHS per day, by provider

Source: Department of Health: *Chief Executives Report to the NHS*, December 2004.

Primary care

Primary care refers to healthcare services provided outside the hospital setting. Central to the NHS, it accounts for 81 per cent of daily patient contacts with the NHS (Figure 4.1), with over 300 million patient contacts each year.[3] It includes the 'family health services' traditionally provided by general practitioners (GPs), dentists, community pharmacists, and opticians. It also includes community health services: i.e. services provided in community settings such as community hospitals and clinics, or in patients' own homes, where they are provided by district nurses or health visitors. Some community health services are also provided by nurses employed by hospitals, but who attend patients at home, such as continence nurses and stomatherapists.

The roles of many of these practitioners are changing, as the DH explores ways to increase the type and level of services provided outside hospital. At the same time a number of alternatives to the traditional providers of primary care are also being developed. These include nurse-led 'walk-in centres' and also NHS Direct, the phone service which will eventually act as the single point of entry to emergency or 'out-of-hours' NHS care.

General practice and the primary healthcare team

GPs are usually people's first point of contact with the NHS. They provide services to patients registered with their practices, generally people who live in the local area. Practices range in size from 'single-handed' GP practices to large medical centres with ten GPs or more. In 2004 there were some 8,944 general practices,[4] with just over 31,500 GPs; when part-time working is taken into account this equates to just over 28,000 'whole-time-equivalent' GPs.[5] As in other areas of the NHS, recruitment of GPs is a continuing problem, with 3,240 GP posts reported vacant in England and Wales in 2003–4.[6]

GPs work alongside other members of the 'primary healthcare team', such as practice nurses, community nurses, health visitors, practice managers and administrative staff.[7] Many of these people, such as practice managers, nurses and receptionists, are employed by GP practices, while others, such as health visitors, are employed centrally by PCTs.[*] They undertake a variety of different roles; receptionists deal with the administration of the practice such as appointments, general enquiries and repeat prescriptions. Practice nurses advise patients with minor illnesses such as colds, as well as performing tasks such as checking blood pressure, dressing wounds, taking blood samples and doing cervical smears. Other members of the team provide community health services. District nurses provide nursing care in the community, such as home visits to elderly patients, and health visitors are responsible for overseeing the health of babies and young

---

* The DH has, however, stated its intention that by December 2008 PCTs will provide services only when these cannot be commissioned or 'purchased' from other providers, and it remains unclear who will provide services such as health visitors.

children. Some practices also have a community midwife who shares with the GP the antenatal care of expectant mothers.

GPs and the primary healthcare team provide what are called 'general medical services' (GMS), treating people who seek medical attention, managing the care of patients with chronic conditions such as respiratory disease, and providing preventative services such as 'health checks' of young babies and mothers. They also act as the 'gatekeepers' who control access to secondary care services, a GP's referral being required for elective or non-emergency access to hospital care; in 2003–4 GPs referred over nine million patients to hospital-based specialists.[8] Since April 2005 GP practices have also been able to hold 'indicative budgets' for commissioning secondary care, and by December 2006 will be responsible for commissioning all aspects of community and secondary healthcare services. As discussed in Chapter 3 (see pages 43–4), this so-called GP-practice based commissioning involves individual practices or groups of practices deciding, within the constraints of their budgets, what secondary and other healthcare services are commissioned or 'purchased' for their patients.

The role of GPs and other members of the primary healthcare team is also being extended through an initiative known as 'practitioners with special interests'. This is intended to improve patient access to more specialist services by moving one million appointments, which would traditionally have taken place in hospital outpatient clinics, into primary care by 2006.[9] It is also intended to bring more secondary care 'procedures', particularly diagnostic tests such as endoscopy and minor surgery, into primary care and community-based settings. This initiative initially focussed on GPs; by May 2004 over 1,300 GPs had developed a 'special interest'[10] and an estimated 532,000 specialist procedures were undertaken in primary care in 2003–4.[11] Nurses and other health professionals such as physiotherapists are also increasingly developing special interests, being employed by PCTs to provide multidisciplinary care for patients with chronic conditions such as diabetes and respiratory disease. This has been facilitated by allowing PCTs to employ health professionals directly to provide specific medical services under arrangements known as 'PCT medical services' (PCTMS); previously PCTs were only able to employ staff to support the provision of medical services through the GMS and PMS arrangements discussed below. The DH intends, however, that by December 2008 PCTs should provide such services only when they cannot be commissioned or 'purchased' from another provider. This means that in the future the provision of such services is unlikely to be undertaken by PCTs.

Unlike the rest of the NHS, where doctors are salaried, GPs are independent practitioners. They operate as small businesses, 'single-handed' or in 'partnerships' of two or more GPs who own or rent their own premises and employ their own staff. Since 2004 the partners can include other members of staff such as practice managers, nurses, allied health professionals and pharmacists. GPs provide their services under contract to their local PCT; in 2005–6 PCTs received £4.5 billion to pay for this.[12] The work is organised in several alternative ways, known respectively as 'general medical services' (GMS), 'personal medical services' (PMS), and salaried GP arrangements.

GPs have traditionally provided services under 'general medical services' or GMS arrangements. In April 2004 a new GMS contract was introduced,* based on locally-negotiated agreements between PCTs and GP practices. Individual GPs are no longer responsible for providing 'comprehensive care' 24 hours a day, seven days a week. Instead, 'essential services', which all practices must provide, are now limited to medical care for those who are ill, or who think they are ill, and the general management of terminally ill patients. Practices can choose whether to provide two further kinds of service: 'additional services', which include chronic disease management, vaccination, contraceptive and child health surveillance services, and which it is assumed practices will normally provide, but which they can 'opt out' of providing; and 'enhanced services', such as minor surgery, which they can 'opt in' to providing.

Furthermore under the new GMS contract GPs are no longer required to provide 'out-of-hours care', defined as services provided from 6.30 pm to 8 am on weekdays, and the whole of weekends, and bank and other public holidays. Practices can choose to provide this care if their PCT agrees, but responsibility for its provision now lies with PCTs. PCTs can provide it through agreements with local practices, or 'co-operatives' of local practices, but can now also contract with 'alternative providers' for the provision of 'specialised services' (such as out-of-hours services) through arrangements known as 'alternative provider medical services' or APMS (see Chapter 3, page 39). Alternative providers may include both 'not for profit' and 'for profit' healthcare organisations, as well as other PCTs (and even NHS hospital trusts and foundation trusts).

The new GMS contract also changed the way GPs are remunerated.† Each practice now receives a practice budget known as the 'global sum' to cover its running costs, which include the GPs' incomes and staff salaries, the provision of essential services, and the costs of providing 'additional services' where they choose to provide these. Further payments are made for providing 'enhanced' primary care services, and practices also receive a sizeable portion of their income in the form of 'quality payments'. These payments are made on the basis of their performance against the 'quality and outcomes framework' (see Chapter 6, page 121), which measures performance against agreed targets in areas relating to clinical, organisational, and patient experience issues, as well as in the provision of additional services. This change in the way GPs are remunerated may seem esoteric, but de-linking remuneration from the number of GPs in a practice has the potential to act as a driver to change the skill-mix in primary care, acting as

* Prior to April 2004 services were provided under terms and conditions of service agreed in 1948 (known as 'the red book'). Individual GPs held contracts with the Secretary of State for Health, which involved responsibility for providing comprehensive care for their patients 24 hours a day, 7 days a week.
† Prior to April 2004 GPs received a payment for each patient on their list, as well as payments for each 'item of service' undertaken and for achieving certain targets such as immunisation rates. These were supplemented by a number of allowances for GP infrastructure such as practice staff, premises, information and technology expenses, costs of administration and GP expenditure on drugs and appliances.

an incentive to reduce the number of GPs in a practice and have more services provided by other, less highly paid, healthcare professionals.

The provision of primary care services under 'personal medical services' or PMS arrangements was introduced in pilot form in April 1998, in an attempt to address ongoing recruitment and retention difficulties and increase the flexibility of service provision, particularly for vulnerable groups such as refugees and asylum seekers. It became a permanent arrangement in 2004, by which time over 37 per cent of GPs were working under PMS contracts.[13]

PMS is a voluntary scheme enabling GP practices to develop their own working arrangements. Locally-negotiated contracts are held between the PCT and the 'PMS scheme', with freedom to negotiate terms and conditions of service for the practitioners, their remuneration, and what services the scheme will provide. To maximise flexibility and innovation in service provision a PCT may hold a PMS contract or contracts with one or more individual GPs, as well as with nurses, dentists and other healthcare professionals employed by a GP practice. For specialist PMS schemes a PCT could also have PMS contracts with staff such as consultants, nurses or allied health professionals employed by the PCT, an NHS trust or a foundation trust.

Under both GMS and PMS arrangements GPs can also now choose to work as salaried GPs, remunerated for working an agreed number of clinical sessions. By 2004, 9 per cent of GPs were salaried.[5]

Alternatives to general practice

Primary care walk-in centres

Primary care walk-in centres were announced in April 1999 as part of the government's commitment to modernise the NHS. These nurse-led centres are intended to improve access to services, acting as a complement to 'mainstream' primary care services by providing open access to advice and treatment for minor injuries and ailments; neither an appointment nor registration with a GP is required. They also provide information about local NHS services, social services and other statutory and voluntary services.

The centres have extended opening hours, typically from early in the morning until late at night seven days a week. While some are located next to existing hospital accident and emergency services (for example Sheffield Royal Hallamshire hospital, or Newham district general hospital), they are also intended to improve geographical access for patients, and particularly for commuters. Thus many are located in town centres (for example in Soho in London) and in transport terminals (such as the walkway between terminals at Manchester airport).

By the end of 2004 there were 65 NHS walk-in centres in England.[14] They are typically run by PCTs, to which they are accountable, with staff employed by the PCT or working under PMS arrangements. The DH's 'suggested' model has a staff pool of 12 whole-time equivalent nursing staff, two receptionists on each shift, and two managerial staff, for an expected 2,500 patients per month.[15] They increasingly also have a GP on site, and many also provide additional services ranging from pharmacy and translating services to mental health services. Over 1.5 million patients attended walk-in centres in the year to April 2004.[16] They have not, however, been shown to significantly reduce the use of other services, such as GP out-of-hours services or accident and emergency departments.[17]

NHS Direct

NHS Direct was introduced in March 1998, and national coverage was achieved by the end of 2000. A nurse-run 24-hour telephone help-line, it is intended to improve the accessibility and responsiveness of services, providing people with easier and faster information and advice about health issues and the NHS. It also provides a 'triaging' system, directing people to the appropriate healthcare provider. Its remit has also been extended, with the aim of making it the sole point of access to out-of-hours care by 2006. To achieve this a series of pilot schemes have begun to address the task of integrating NHS Direct with mainstream providers of out-of-hours care, including general practice out-of-hours services, low priority emergency ambulance calls, and accident and emergency departments. An associated on-line service (offering all but the triaging service) was launched in December 1999, and it is intended that a digital TV service providing information and advice will also become available.

NHS Direct is now the world's largest provider of telephone health advice, receiving 6.4 million calls, and 6.5 million visits to its online services, in 2003–4.[16] In April 2004 it was made into a special health authority, as a 'national provider unit' responsible for delivering services across the country through 22 regional provider units. With 2,000 staff, many of them recruited from other NHS organisations, by 2005–6 it had operating costs of £163 million,[18] the necessary funds being allocated on a capitation or population basis to PCTs which commission or 'purchase' its services. It is to remain as a national service, but within the next two to three years it will cease to be a special health authority and will be given some kind of independent status – as a non-profit 'public interest company, an 'alternative' commercial model (such as a limited liability partnership with the government), a corporate body, a charity, or an NHS foundation trust.

Since April 2004 PCTs have thus been responsible for commissioning or 'purchasing' NHS Direct services on behalf of their local populations. The DH intends that this should in the future be undertaken by consortia of PCTs, in order to achieve economies. NHS Direct services are commissioned using a framework similar to that of the new GMS contract discussed above (page 51). They are categorised into three levels. The first level is 'nationally directed services', consisting of the telephone help-line service which offers general health information and advice as well as suggesting the most appropriate referral for specific clinical problems; the NHS Direct website offering information and advice on general health issues; the intended digital TV service; and the provision of support in the event of a major incident, such as providing a telephone help-line service. Nationally-directed services are those which are currently commissioned by PCTs on a capitation basis, paying NHS Direct a set amount per head of population, although the intention is to move towards a set cost per call.

The second category is 'nationally enhanced services'. This includes the development by December 2006 of NHS Direct as the single point of access to emergency or 'out-of-hours' services: people will have to go through NHS Direct to gain access to an out-of-hours GP. As part of this remit it is also intended that NHS Direct will manage low-priority ambulance calls, and provide telephone interpreting and translation services to which every NHS organisation will have access. 'Nationally enhanced services' are commissioned by PCTs on an activity basis; they pay NHS Direct for the number of calls their residents make to it.

The third category is 'locally enhanced services', which PCTs can commission or 'purchase' according to local needs. Examples include the use of NHS Direct infra-structure and information on the NHS and local services to train staff for Patient Advice and Liaison Services or PALS (see Chapter 6, page 130), or the provision of call handling services, such as rapid response lines for NHS trusts following major incidents.

As a special health authority NHS Direct is accountable to the Secretary of State for Health and is subject to the general corporate governance arrangements of the NHS. Thus it has a board with both executive and non-executive directors and a lay chair, who are accountable for the quality of its services and its effective use of funds. NHS Direct is also accountable to the PCTs which commission (or 'purchase') its services, through its contracts with them, which should specify the nature and quality of the services to be provided. Like other NHS bodies it is subject to a duty of clinical governance (see Chapter 6, pages 114–16), being required to put into place systems and processes to ensure the quality of the services provided. These include measures such as the regular audit of services, the education and development of staff, the use of evidence-based practice, a risk-management framework, and the monitoring and reviewing of complaints, professional feedback and adverse incidents. When NHS Direct achieves independent status (as a commercial company or a foundation trust, for example) it will fall outside the NHS requirements for corporate and clinical governance and will then be accountable only through its contracts with PCTs, and perhaps to Monitor (see Chapter 6, pages 108–13).

Non-NHS primary care

Historically the NHS has provided more or less universal primary care services which are free at the point of use, and GPs are not allowed to treat patients privately if they are registered with them under the NHS. For these reasons the private provision of primary care services has traditionally been small, accounting for only 3 per cent of all GP consultations in Britain.[19]

These are provided by a small number of GPs (around 200) most of whom practise exclusively privately, providing services to wealthy patients, particularly in the London area.[20] A number of GPs also provide 'part time' private services by working, for part of their time, for companies that provide primary care services.

As part of an emerging 'market' in primary care services (which has been described aptly as 'embryonic')[20] these services are mainly targeted at professionals and the corporate sector in London. Services are provided either on a fee-per-consultation basis or through yearly subscription plans. Different models of service provision include private walk-in medical centres run by companies such as General Medical Clinics plc and the Franbar group (which owns Medicentres UK); private general practices located on private hospital sites; company-paid private GP services for employees, such as those insured by BUPA: and private capitation schemes in which patients pay a set annual sum to a company which employs GPs to treat them.

The provision of private primary care services is, however, set to rise. Since the introduction of the new GP contract in 2004 PCTs are now responsible for securing the full range of primary care services for their populations, while GPs can decide not to provide certain elements of these services, for both in-hours and out-of-hours services. PCTs are being encouraged to be more innovative in how they get them provided, and are now able to commission or 'purchase' them from the independent sector through the new APMS (alternative provider medical services) arrangements mentioned earlier (Nestor Healthcare plc has been mentioned, for example, as wishing to develop services to be provided to the NHS on a contract basis).[21] PCTs are also able to provide services directly themselves through the new PCTMS (PCT medical services) arrangements (described above, page 50), and some authors have proposed that PCTs could generate revenue by selling primary care services to private patients.[20]

Other family health services

In addition to services provided through general practices, other elements of family health services are provided by dentists, opticians and community pharmacists. These are provided under contracts with the local PCT , which holds a list of local practitioners registered to provide NHS services.

NHS dentistry

All treatment necessary to maintain oral health is, or should be, available on the NHS. Unlike other NHS treatments, however, it is not 'free at the point of delivery'. Patients are liable for most of a prescribed fee for every course of treatment, although some groups, such as children, pregnant women, and those on income support are exempt from fees. Adults currently pay 80 per cent of the cost of treatment up to a maximum of £378 per course of treatment.[22] In 2004 the NHS provided dental services through some 19,300 dentists.[23] In 2002–3 almost 17 million adults and seven million children were registered with NHS dentists, and adults received over 26 million courses of NHS treatment.[24]

Responsibility for securing NHS dental services was devolved to PCTs in October 2005, under the 2003 Health and Social Care (Community Health and Standards) Act. PCTs now hold the budget for providing dental services, at an estimated cost (net of patient charges) in 2005–6 of £1.6 billion.[25] They are responsible both for assessing the local need for services and for securing their provision, which they do through contracts with qualified dental practitioners who are registered with the General Dental Council, according to a national framework agreement.

NHS dental services have traditionally been provided under an arrangement known as 'general dental services' or GDS, whereby dentists have individual contracts to provide NHS services. With the introduction of a new GDS contract in October 2005, however, the aim is to move towards PCTs making contracts with dental practices rather than with individual dentists. This new contract has also changed the system of remuneration for NHS dental services, moving from a 'fee for service' system, whereby dentists were paid for each item of work, to a system where practices receive an annual amount with which to provide dental care to their patients. This is paid in monthly instalments by the Business Services Authority (see Chapter 2, page 25).

Dentists operate as independent practitioners and so are free to choose whether to provide NHS services at all; if they do they are required to provide them only for patients registered with their practice through the NHS. While most dental practices take both private and NHS patients, the proportion of dentists' time spent treating NHS patients has fallen, with a severe undersupply of NHS dentists in many areas. Indeed the shortfall of 1,850 practising dentists (both NHS and non-NHS) in 2004 was projected to rise to a shortfall of 5,100 whole-time equivalents by 2011. These issues are being addressed through the recruitment of dentists from abroad and attempts to increase the NHS commitment of existing dentists. Plans assume that an expanded NHS dental workforce will be able to treat two million more patients by 2005–6.[24]

Initiatives to increase the provision of NHS dental services include allowing PCTs to employ dental healthcare professionals directly, using locally-negotiated personal dental services (PDS) arrangements. These are flexible arrangements introduced in 1998 to address problems of local supply, analogous to PMS arrangements for general medical services (see page 52 above). By 2004, 3,500 dentists were working under PDS arrangements in 1,300 practices.[26] Another initiative was the introduction in 2000 of dental 'open access' centres: by 2004 there were 47 such centres operating in areas with the worst access problems.[27] The centres provide urgent NHS care for patients who are not registered with a dental practice. Depending on the centre, they also offer routine care, or will help patients to find a local dental practice with which to register. Meanwhile the law is also being changed to allow much greater provision of NHS dental services by private companies.*

---

* Under the 1956 Dentists Act corporate bodies are barred from providing NHS dental services, only the 28 in operation at the time of the Act being allowed to continue to do so.

NHS ophthalmic services

The NHS provides 'general ophthalmic services' or GOS in the form of free sight tests for children and for people aged over 60, as well as for people with certain eye conditions or in receipt of benefits such as income support. Children, people with complex lens prescriptions, and people receiving certain benefits such as income support also receive NHS vouchers towards the cost of glasses. These services are provided by ophthalmic practitioners, i.e. qualified practitioners registered with the General Optical Council to test eyesight and prescribe and dispense glasses. They provide services under contract with PCTs and are reimbursed according to a national fee schedule. PCTs hold and govern the list of local practitioners registered to provide NHS ophthalmic services.

In 2004 there were 8,331 ophthalmic practitioners under contract to provide NHS sight tests, operating in over 6,000 establishments, mainly in 'high-street' locations.[28] They include smaller independent practitioners as well as large corporations such as Boots and Vision Express. Ophthalmic practitioners are primarily optometrists (also known as opticians), but they also include a small number of ophthalmic medical practitioners (qualified doctors who specialise in eye care and are qualified to test eyesight and prescribe spectacles). Expenditure on general ophthalmic services was £322 million in 2003–4, when ophthalmic practitioners carried out 9.8 million NHS sight tests and claimed reimbursement for optical vouchers towards 3.5 million pairs of glasses.[27]

As with other elements of family health services the DH is examining ways to extend the role of primary care ophthalmic services to provide more specialist care outside hospitals. This includes PCTs developing 'shared care' schemes, to facilitate closer working between optometrists and hospital ophthalmologists. For example optometrists may screen for conditions such as glaucoma or diabetic eye disease, and refer patients to hospital ophthalmologists using agreed referral protocols.

NHS pharmaceutical services

NHS pharmaceutical services within primary care consist of the dispensing of NHS prescriptions for drugs, medicines, and appliances such as syringes or devices to monitor blood glucose levels. Prescriptions are written by GPs and dentists, and also, since 2003, by nurses and pharmacists qualifying as 'supplementary prescribers' who are able to prescribe a limited range of prescription-only medicines. The actual dispensing of prescriptions is undertaken by community pharmacists, and in rural areas by GP surgeries.

Almost 10,000 pharmacies have contracts to dispense NHS prescriptions,[29] and 75 per cent of GP surgeries have a community pharmacy within 300 metres.[30] These include smaller independent pharmacists as well as large corporations such as Boots; the top three companies (Lloyds, Boots and Moss) have 28 per cent of the market.[31] In the year to June 2004, 668 million prescriptions were dispensed, the drugs themselves costing £7.8 billion. This represents an increase of 128 million prescriptions (a 24 per cent increase) and £2.3 billion in drug costs (a 41 per cent increase) since *The NHS Plan* was published in the year 2000.[32]

Most NHS adult patients pay a standard charge for prescriptions (£6.50 since April 2005); but children, those aged over 60, and those in receipt of benefits such as income support and sickness benefit, are exempt from charges, and account for the great majority of all prescriptions issued (over the years 1999–2004 the percentage remained fairly constant at 85 per cent).[33] Pharmacists and GP practices which dispense drugs are reimbursed on behalf of PCTs by the Business Services Authority (see Chapter 2, page 25). They are reimbursed for the cost of the drug or appliance plus a professional fee or allowance, according to a schedule laid out in the Drug Tariff, produced monthly by the Business Services Authority on behalf of the Secretary of State.

Community pharmacies provide their services under contract to their PCT. Pharmacies apply to PCTs to provide services in accordance with a statutory scheme, with terms of service set out in regulations. A new contractual framework was introduced in April 2005, again analogous to the GMS contract for GPs. Thus all pharmacists providing NHS services are required to provide nationally defined 'essential services', which include dispensing pharmaceuticals, 'repeat dispensing',* disposing of returned or unused medicines, the promotion of healthy lifestyles (particularly among those at risk, such as diabetics, those with high blood pressure and those who are overweight), advice on self-care for patients with minor or chronic illness, and 'sign-posting' patients to other healthcare services. Pharmacists can also choose to gain accreditation to provide various 'advanced' services, such as undertaking 'medicines reviews'.† PCTs can also commission locally-determined 'enhanced' services from community pharmacists, according to the needs of the local population. Examples include pharmacists providing smoking cessation services, services and support to residents in care homes, and acting as 'supplementary prescribers' with the ability to prescribe a limited number of medicines. Prior to the implementation of the new contracting framework pharmacies are providing such services through 'local pharmaceutical services' (LPS) arrangements.

PCTs hold and govern entry to the list of local pharmacies that are registered to provide NHS services. The regulations governing entry of pharmacies to this list are being changed, along with the new contractual framework for the delivery of services. The DH's intention is to 'maintain and improve access to pharmacists in all communities', but at the same time to 'move cautiously in the direction recommended by the OFT' (the Office of Fair Trading) ‡, towards a deregulated system of pharmaceutical services.[34] This involves PCTs considering applications

---

* Under repeat dispensing patients are given sufficient prescription forms to enable pharmacists to keep dispensing their prescriptions for up to a year without seeing a doctor again.

† Medicines reviews are periodic systematic discussions with patients to check their compliance with their prescribed treatments and discuss any problems they may have with their medicines.

‡ In 2003 an OFT report on *The Control of Entry Regulations and Retail Pharmacy Services in the UK* (London: OFT) recommended the deregulation of pharmaceutical services, ending control over which pharmacists could dispense NHS prescriptions.

from new providers, notably large private pharmacy chains, so as to increase competition and choice. The presumption is now that new applications to join the list are accepted unless they are considered by the PCT to be clearly detrimental to the adequate provision of pharmaceutical services in the neighbourhood.*

Certain categories of providers are also entirely exempt from PCTs' control of entry to their lists, namely pharmacies in large 'out of town' shopping developments, pharmacies opening more than 100 hours per week, pharmacies established as part of 'one stop shops'† offering a wide range of community-based services to populations of over 18,000 patients, and internet or mail order-based services providing fully professional services.

Community health services

Community health services are healthcare services provided in community settings, such as community hospitals, hospices, health centres and patients' homes. They are provided by a number of different NHS organisations. For example a number of NHS (hospital) trusts and PCTs also run community hospitals, providing services such as physiotherapy, rehabilitation, and residential care for older and disabled people. As previously noted, however, the DH intends that by December 2008 PCTs should provide such services only when they cannot be commissioned or 'purchased' from another provider. This means that their role in the provision of community health services will be reduced. This is intended to encourage the use and development of 'alternative' providers of community health services, in turn encouraging the development of 'contestability' or competition in such services.

There are also 13 community trusts which provide such services, as well as eight care trusts and 45 specialist mental health trusts.[35] These three kinds of trust typically provide nurses and 'outreach' teams to provide continuing care and therapy in community settings, while stomatherapy, breast cancer nursing and specialist services for conditions such as diabetes or incontinence are provided in the community by nurses from NHS (hospital) trusts. In 2003–4 such nurses provided care to over 260,000 people. Community health services are also provided by members of the primary health care team, such as district nurses and health visitors. In 2003–4 two million people received care in their own homes, such as the dressing of wounds, from district nurses,[36] while three million people, 62 per cent of whom were children aged under five, received care from health visitors.[37]

The important role played by community health services has been recognised in the DH's policy of supporting people with chronic conditions to live healthy lives. By 2008 it is intended that 'community matrons' will provide case management for vulnerable patients (people with three or more long-term health problems). As specialist clinicians (often nurses), community matrons will liaise with GPs and

---

* At issue is whether existing, usually small, neighborhood pharmacies may be put out of business by new outlets of the big pharmacy chains, reducing access for some patients.

† 'One stop shop' primary care centres bring together a range of primary, community, and social care services on one site.

primary care teams to develop individual care plans for their patients. By 2008 it is intended that over 3,000 community matrons will be providing such care for 250,000 patients.[38]

Since April 2003 the NHS has been responsible for providing free nursing (as opposed to personal) care for all those living in the community, irrespective of their type of residence. In 2004–5, 1.3 million people were eligible for nursing care in community settings, and PCTs were allocated £600 million to fund it.[39]

Social care services for adults are predominantly commissioned by local authorities from 'independent sector' (voluntary or for-profit) providers;* in 2002–3, 64 per cent of the contact hours of home help or home care, and 79 per cent of placements in residential care homes, were commissioned from the independent sector.[40] Total funding for personal social services in England in 2005–6 has been set at £14.6 billion. £2.1 billion of this will come from the DH.[41] †

Secondary care

Secondary care has historically consisted of the provision of specialised services, both inpatient and outpatient, in a hospital setting. It encompasses medical specialties such as dermatology and cardiology, surgical specialties such as urology and orthopaedics, as well as age-defined specialties such as paediatrics and elderly care. Patients are generally under the care of a consultant (senior hospital doctor), and unless they are admitted via the accident and emergency department they require a referral from a GP. A number of hospitals also provide highly specialised tertiary services, such as neuro-surgery, thoracic surgery and haemophilia services. Often requiring sophisticated equipment and support facilities, these services are provided to larger catchment populations of over one million people,[42] and referral has to come from a hospital consultant rather than a GP.

As we saw earlier (page 48), hospitals account for over 50 per cent of the budget for NHS service provision[41] but only 19 per cent of the daily contacts with the NHS,[42] and the development of alternatives to hospital-based secondary

---

* The non-nursing elements of the care required to enable vulnerable people, such as the elderly or those with physical or learning disabilities, to carry out the activities of daily living, are the responsibility of local authority social services departments, and are charged for, subject to means-testing. Termed 'personal social services' or 'social care', they include services such as the provision of equipment and home adaptations, help with washing and dressing, attendance at day centres, and supported accommodation in residential and nursing homes. In 2002–3, 1.4 million people received some form of home care, while in 2003–4 over 3 million contact hours of social care were provided in people's own homes, with 87,000 households receiving 'intensive' care (defined as more than ten contact hours and more than six visits per week). Long term supported care is provided in residential and nursing homes; 370,000 adults were in such placements in 2002–3.

† As described in Chapter 2 (pages 12 and 14) the DH oversees the 'personal social services' provided by local authorities. The publicly funded share of the cost of providing these services is partly provided by the DH, though from outside the NHS budget.

care has been a key policy aim of the DH. Initiatives to achieve this include the development of primary care professionals with special interests (discussed above on page 50), who are able to provide specialist services in primary care settings. At the same time alternatives to NHS hospital trusts are being developed, with the introduction of foundation trusts, the establishment of treatment centres providing 'stand-alone' elective services, and the introduction of independent sector (for-profit and voluntary) providers as mainstream providers of secondary care for the NHS. Key to this agenda is enabling patients to choose their providers of elective services. From December 2005 patients requiring an elective procedure should be able to choose, in discussion with their GP, from four to five possible providers,[43] and by 2008 they will have the right to choose from any provider, including any independent sector provider, which meets NHS standards and will provide the treatment at NHS prices (the national tariff described in Chapter 5, pages 97–8).

NHS hospital trusts

Establishment

NHS hospitals were established as autonomous bodies known as 'trusts' under the 1990 NHS and Community Care Act, and by 1996 all district general and specialist hospitals had achieved trust status. The 1999 Health Act, however, brought them back under the control of the Secretary of State for Health, so that although they continue to function as legally independent bodies, the Secretary of State has the power to direct them in the exercise of their functions.

By 2005 there were 153 'acute' NHS trusts providing hospital services, and a further 20 providing purely specialist or tertiary services.[*][44] Between them they provide over 100,000 hospital beds.[45] Due to mergers and acquisitions many trusts provide services on more than one hospital and/or community site; for example Newcastle upon Tyne Hospitals NHS trust provides services from four hospital sites, plus a dental hospital and a fertility and genetics centre. Some, however, like Hereford Hospital NHS trust, provide services from a single site.

Function

NHS trusts provide acute (emergency) and elective (planned) secondary care services; there were 9.9 million admissions to NHS trusts in England in 2004–5, 45 per cent of which were for emergency care and 55 per cent for elective care.[46] There were 16.7 million new attendances at A and E. Some trusts also provide community health services.

NHS trusts earn most of their income by 'selling' their services to PCTs, and since April 2005 also to GP practice-based commissioners (see Chapter 3,

---

* There were also 83 trusts (including some of those already mentioned) providing specialist mental health services, three providing learning disability services, and 31 providing ambulance services.

pages 43–4). These commissions are based on NHS contracts, which are not legally binding but which are overseen and can be enforced by the Secretary of State for Health. PCTs and GP practice-based commissioners commission these services on behalf of their populations or registered patients, which meant that until December 2005 trusts provided services to the geographically-defined population of their local PCTs and/or GP practices. The introduction of the choice initiative, however, is changing the populations to whom NHS trusts provide services. Depending on how patients exercise their new right to choose their own provider of elective services, NHS trusts may find themselves increasingly providing services to patients from geographically distant locations. Some NHS trusts, moreover, have already seen the marketing of their services to overseas patients as playing an important part in securing their future revenue.

NHS trusts are also able to 'earn' income by charging for services they provide to non-NHS patients, i.e. 'self-paying' or 'company-paid' private patients from the UK and overseas. In 2003–4 income from private patients was expected to generate £408 million for NHS trusts in the UK as a whole. In England this accounts for 1.1 per cent of trusts' core revenue; the proportion is lower in the devolved countries (0.3 per cent in Wales and Northern Ireland, and 0.1 per cent in Scotland).[47] These services are concentrated in 'private patient units', dedicated wards or wings within NHS hospitals which often also have dedicated staff and operating theatre facilities. In mid-2004 there were 79 such units with 1,275 beds in the UK as a whole. Twenty two of these units, and 531 of the beds, are in the greater London area, and eight of the ten trusts with the highest private revenues are in central London. The highest earner is the Royal Marsden Hospital trust, which provides oncology services and receives almost a quarter of its patient-activity income from private patients.[48]

NHS trusts can also sub-contract work to other providers, predominantly in the independent sector. In the year 2001–2 (the latest year for which data are available) this was done mainly to tackle waiting list priorities; 46,000 procedures were sub-contracted, mainly for cataracts, hip and knee replacements, hernia repairs, and varicose veins, at a cost of £91 million.[49] The number has greatly increased since then. Some NHS trusts also sub-contract diagnostic services such as radiology and pathology services to independent-sector providers; on the other hand some NHS trusts 'sell' such services to independent-sector hospitals.

NHS trusts are required to work in partnership with other NHS bodies and local authorities, and are required to produce annual plans detailing how they will achieve national and local priorities and fit within the plans of their PCT commissioners. With a policy emphasis on integration within the local NHS it is intended that they will deliver services through 'clinical networks' made up of all the organisations involved in managing the care of patients with particular conditions.

In addition to their freedom to generate income by such measures as leasing space in their foyers to companies like McDonalds, and charging for car parking, NHS trusts are also intended to use the power provided by the 2001 Health and Social Care Act to undertake joint ventures with the independent (private and voluntary) sector to generate additional income. This possibility includes establishing companies to provide healthcare services and to exploit intellectual property rights, for instance by marketing the findings of research studies and technological advances.

Structure

NHS trusts are corporate bodies, governed by boards of directors which oversee their work and strategic direction and ensure that they meet key DH objectives such as waiting-time targets. The boards are also collectively responsible for ensuring that trusts meet their financial, statutory, and legal responsibilities. Board membership is limited to 11, with up to five executive directors who oversee the day-to-day running of the trust's activities. The membership must include the chief executive, the finance director, the medical director and the director of nursing. The board has a 'lay' chair and five non-executive directors appointed by the NHS Appointments Commission (see Chapter 2, pages 31–2); these members are intended to give representation to the population served by the trust.

Higher-performing NHS trusts (as determined by the Healthcare Commission – see Chapter 6, pages 116–20) are allowed to set their own management costs, following consultation with their clinicians. Other NHS trusts are required to keep their management costs within NHS Plan targets, and are overseen in this regard by their Strategic Health Authority or SHA. For 2005–6 the annual increase in management costs for a trust should be less than the annual rate of increase in NHS expenditure (7.2 per cent for 2003–4).[50] The latest figures, for 2002–3, show that management costs for NHS trusts in England were £1.3 billion.[51]

Foundation trusts

Establishment

The concept of foundation trusts (FTs) was introduced in the 2002 government publication, *Delivering the NHS Plan*. They were subsequently legislated for in the 2003 NHS Health and Social Care (Community Health and Standards) Act, which enabled NHS organisations to be established as 'public benefit corporations' known as FTs.

Since April 2004 high-performing or 'very good' NHS trusts in England, as determined by the Healthcare Commission, have been able to apply for foundation status. Such trusts must first ask the Secretary of State for Health for approval to apply to the independent regulator, Monitor. Monitor, already described in Chapter 2 (page 30) and discussed more fully in Chapter 6 (pages 112–13), authorises foundation status by providing trusts with 'terms of authorisation', in effect a licence to operate. By September 2005, 31 NHS trusts had been granted foundation status,[52] and 32 more had been granted approval to apply in the next round of applications.[53] The DH intends that all NHS trusts should achieve foundation status by 2008, and supports this aim with a £200 million investment programme to help trusts achieve the required level of performance.[54]

The 2003 Health and Social Care (Community Health and Standards) Act also allows Monitor to authorise other bodies to become foundation trusts. This has not yet happened but could include NHS bodies such as PCTs and care trusts (see Chapter 3, pages 36–43 and 44–6), as well as non-NHS organisations such as voluntary and for-profit health care providers.

Function

The function of FTs is to provide goods and services on behalf of the health service in England. Their licences to operate stipulate the goods and services they are required to supply on behalf of the NHS, such as numbers of inpatient admissions and day-case and outpatient attendances for different specialties. Like other NHS bodies they are required to co-operate with other NHS and partner organisations to deliver these services. They must also provide for the ongoing education and training of staff, and participate in wider NHS activities such as research and development.

Their duties, however, are otherwise limited to a requirement to exercise their functions 'effectively, efficiently and economically,'[55] and they have a number of important differences and freedoms compared with NHS trusts. They are free from the direction of the Secretary of State for Health and able to determine their own priorities for service provision and development, developing services on the basis of the demand for them rather than on the basis of national priorities determined by the Secretary of State. FTs are also freed from 'performance management' by their local SHA (see Chapter 6, pages 108–9). Their performance is supervised instead by the independent regulator, Monitor, in terms of how well they conform to the terms of their licences to operate (Chapter 6, pages 112–13).

Unlike the contracts used for NHS trusts, FTs provide their services to PCTs on the basis of legally binding contracts. They are also free to provide private health services; although the proportion of their income (as opposed to the total amount) that they can earn from this source is capped, the cap is under review.* Unlike other NHS bodies FTs are free to dispose of (i.e. sell) 'unprotected assets', namely land and buildings that are not required for the provision of NHS 'mandatory' services, and they can also dispose of 'protected assets' (those used for the provision of NHS services) if they have the approval of Monitor. Subject to Monitor's approval they can also retain all the proceeds,† either to reinvest in their services or to use as security for borrowing.

FTs can apply to their SHA for NHS funds to support capital investment, but unlike NHS trusts they can also borrow from the private sector for this purpose,

---

*   The income FTs may earn from the provision of private health care is capped at the proportion they earned from this source in their first year as foundation trusts.
†   NHS trusts, by contrast, can only retain up to a maximum of £10 million of the proceeds from asset sales, the amount depending on their turnover and on their performance rating from the Healthcare Commission. Department of Health, *New Delegated Limits for Capital Investment: 2003*, online at <http://www.dh.gov.uk/assetRoot/04/05/66/83/04056683.pdf> (Accessed 3 September 2005).

following a 'prudential code' or limit determined by Monitor. An FT's ability to service debt determines its ability to achieve a credit rating, the possession of which enables it to borrow on commercial terms. FTs may also undertake joint ventures with the independent (for-profit or voluntary) sector. This enables them to enter into commercial and non-commercial ventures in order to raise income, and these ventures need not be related to healthcare.

Structure

FTs are independent 'public benefit' corporations, not-for-profit companies which re-invest any profits in services rather than distributing them to shareholders. Subject to certain constraints they are free to determine their own governance arrangements, which unlike other NHS organisations include, in addition to a board of directors, 'members' and a board of governors. These arrangements are set out by each FT in a 'constitution' approved by Monitor.

THE BOARD OF DIRECTORS

Like NHS trusts FTs are corporate bodies. Each has a board of directors which oversees its strategic direction, and is responsible for ensuring that it meets its financial responsibilities and delivers services in accordance with its licence to operate, overseeing the utilisation of funds and the provision of services. Few requirements relating to the structure of FT boards are laid down, except that they must have at least four executive directors; they may have any number of non-executive or 'lay' directors, one of whom must also be the chair of the board. The executive directors, who are responsible, with the senior management team, for overseeing the day-to day-running of the FT, must include the chief executive, the finance director, a medical or dental practitioner and a nursing or mid-wife practitioner. The non-executive directors must be drawn from the population served by the FT (the FT's 'public constituency'), or be former or current patients of the FT (its 'patient constituency'); and unlike the directors of NHS trusts, who are appointed by the NHS Appointments Commission, the non-executive directors of FTs are appointed by boards of governors who are in turn elected by the FT's 'members'.

MEMBERS AND BOARDS OF GOVERNORS

FTs are the only NHS organisations to have 'members' and elected boards of governors. These are intended to increase the influence of the public, patients and hospital staff in the management of FTs, and to increase the accountability of FTs to them. 'Membership' is open to all local residents of the area to which the FT provides services (the FT's 'public constituency', defined by local authority electoral ward boundaries); to past and current patients of the FT (the 'patient constituency'); and to current staff who have worked in the FT for more than 12 months (the 'staff constituency'). The general rule is that any eligible person can become a member by simply applying; some FTs, however, operate an 'opt-out' system, under which patients and staff automatically become members unless they explicitly decline to be. The members are supposed to be representative of the local community. They may stand for election to the board of governors, and vote in elections for governors; and they should be consulted on matters relating to the provision of services. As of August 2004, 256,860 people were 'members' of the first 20 FTs. Membership ranged from 1,506 members at the Royal Marsden FT in London to 96,174 members at the University Hospital Birmingham FT.[55]

The board of governors of an FT cannot veto decisions of the board of directors, but it may influence policy through its power to appoint the chair of the board of directors and other non-executive directors. They are expected to 'work with' the board of directors to ensure that the FT meets its terms of authorisation, and are required to report to Monitor any concerns they may have regarding the board of directors or the senior management team. The board of governors is also responsible for feeding information about the FTs performance back to the members of the 'constituencies' it represents.

Each FT determines the size and exact constitution of its board of governors. In the first group or 'wave' of FTs to be authorised the numbers of governors varied; for example City Hospitals in Sunderland NHS FT had 19, whilst Basildon and Thurrock University Hospitals NHS FT had 53.[56] The only requirement is that a majority of governors must be elected by the FT's members in its public, patients and staff constituencies. At least three of the governors must be elected by the staff members. There was an overall turnout for elections of 36 per cent: 53 per cent of the public constituencies, 27 per cent of the patient constituencies, and 26 per cent of the staff constituencies.[56] At least one governor should be appointed to represent the PCTs commissioning the FT's services, and at least one should represent the local authorities in the area. Other partner organisations, such as medical or dental schools, may also each be represented by a governor.

Treatment centres

Establishment

Following the examples of European 'polyclinics', and day surgery centres in the USA, 'treatment centres' were introduced into the NHS in 1999 with the opening of an ambulatory care and day-case unit at the Central Middlesex Hospital in London. Subsequently recognised within *The NHS Plan,* they have become a key feature of the government's attempts to 'modernise' the NHS. By the spring of 2005 there were 32 NHS treatment centres providing services, and a further 14 in development.[57] Acquiring additional capacity from independent sector treatment centres (ISTCs) has also become a key government policy. The DH is managing a centrally-run procurement programme, with independent sector providers (in this instance for-profit rather than voluntary) bidding to provide treatment centres in ten local projects, as well as through nine national and regional chains.[58]

Function

Treatment centres carry out planned or 'elective' work, both diagnostic and therapeutic, in separate premises and with separate staff from emergency care (to avoid planned procedures being cancelled to make way for emergencies). They also increase the number of elective procedures which can be performed as day-cases or 'short stay' cases, reducing the need for hospital admissions. They focus on providing high volumes of low-risk procedures in the specialties in which waiting times are particularly long, such as orthopaedics and ophthalmology.

The government's target for treatment centres was that they should provide at least 250,000 'additional' procedures a year by December 2005, 144,000 of them in NHS treatment centres and 106,000 in ISTCs.[59] Although treatment centres are said to be providing 'additional' procedures, in some instances they are replacing work previously carried out in NHS trusts. For example King's College Hospital NHS trust in London now delivers 70 per cent of its elective surgical procedures in its own specialist treatment centre.[60]

Treatment centres are intended to be stand-alone provider units, with PCTs commissioning or 'purchasing' services from them separately, even when they are owned by an NHS trust, using the new financial framework outlined in Chapter 5 (pages 96–9). For treatment centres run by NHS trusts this involves NHS contracts which are not enforceable at law, though overseen by the Secretary of State for Health; in the case of ISTCs the contracts are legally binding, and of five years' duration.

Structure

Treatment centres are situated either within existing hospitals or at independent sites. The independent sector also offers less traditional methods of providing care: for example in February 2004 'Netcare' began operating a mobile treatment centre providing cataract services, performing an average of 39 cataract removals a day in various locations.[61]

A variety of organisations may run treatment centres: PCTs, NHS trusts, joint ventures between the NHS and independent sector, and independent sector providers. The latter include UK-based corporations such as Care UK Afro, as well as international providers such as Anglo-Canadian. The DH is encouraging both UK and international independent healthcare providers to bring overseas medical staff to work in ISTCs in England. Along with the recruitment of overseas medical staff to work in NHS treatment centres this is seen as a way of overcoming NHS capacity constraints due to staff shortages. NHS staff can, however, also work in independent sector treatment centres, for example on a secondment basis.

The independent sector

Establishment

Although the independent sector, which encompasses both voluntary and private organisations, has always delivered some secondary care services on behalf of the NHS, these have traditionally been on a small scale. Until 2000 NHS commissioners purchasing secondary care services were under direction from the DH to do so only when absolutely necessary, using 'spot purchasing' to supplement mainstream provision by NHS providers, for example to ease capacity constraints so as to be able to continue to perform planned, elective procedures during winter periods of peak demand. A number of NHS trusts also used the independent sector to help them meet waiting-list targets by sub-contracting out elective procedures in areas such as ophthalmology and orthopaedics.

In 2000, however, *The NHS Plan* outlined a new relationship between the NHS and the independent sector, intended to make the independent sector a mainstream provider of elective secondary care services for the NHS. The independent sector was also to become a mainstream provider of 'intermediate care' services for the elderly, a form of 'step-down' care provided for elderly people who leave secondary care but are not yet sufficiently well to return home. This was followed in October 2000 by a 'concordat' between the DH and the independent sector, enabling PCTs to commission all forms of care from private and voluntary providers, albeit with an emphasis on elective procedures. Subsequently described by the Secretary of State for Health as 'a permanent feature of the new NHS landscape',[62] the independent sector is seen as providing a means to increase capacity in service provision and increase patients' choice of providers, becoming in effect a component of mainstream provision under NHS auspices.

Function

The independent sector generates most of its revenue from acute or secondary care medical and surgical work, for both inpatients and outpatients. In 2003–4 this amounted to just under £2.2 billion in the UK as a whole.[*63] Most of its hospital admissions are for discrete 'minor' or 'intermediate' surgical procedures, over 80 per cent being for procedures such as endoscopies, cataracts, joint replacement, termination of pregnancies and hernia repairs.[64] In 2003–4 it was estimated that only 9 per cent of its revenue from inpatient, outpatient and day-cases was funded by the NHS; 67 per cent was funded by private medical insurance and the remainder by self-paying UK and overseas patients.[65]

The independent sector was introduced as a mainstream provider of NHS services to help increase capacity in the provision of discrete elective procedures

---

*   The private sector also generates a smaller amount of revenue by providing services not funded or poorly provided by the NHS; in 2003–4 it earned £537 million from psychiatric services, including rehabilitation and substance dependency treatments, as well as £4 million from fertility treatments.

and diagnostic techniques, especially for specialties in which waiting times were long. For example in 2004–5 the DH commissioned 25,000 orthopaedic procedures from the independent sector through a central initiative, largely to address waiting-list problems.[66] The direct commissioning or 'purchasing' of independent sector services by PCTs has also increased considerably since the 'concordat' of 2000. It was estimated that 85,000 NHS patients were treated in the independent sector across the UK in 2003–4, predominantly for procedures such as cataracts and hip and knee replacements.[67] This compared with 6.7 million operations in NHS hospitals,[68] and represented only 1.25 per cent of the total number of operations in that year.

The DH expects, however, that by 2008 the independent sector will be carrying out up to 15 per cent of NHS procedures every year.[69] This will include the provision of services as a result of patient choice, since for elective procedures 'ultimately patients will be able to choose any provider that can meet NHS standards at the NHS tariff'.[70] * Thus PCTS, and in the future GP-practice based commissioners, will commission or 'purchase' 'mainstream' NHS services from independent sector providers. Unlike the commissioning of services from NHS trusts, this will be based upon the use of legally binding contracts, enforceable by law.

Independent sector providers have also acquired a further role within the NHS. Along with high-performing NHS trusts (as determined by the Healthcare Commission – see Chapter 6, pages 116–20) they can apply to be placed on the DH's 'register of expertise', which allows them to bid for the 'franchise' or management of persistently 'failing' NHS trusts or PCTs (see Chapter 6, page 120). The register, established in 2002, contains eight independent sector commercial companies[†] as well as 62 NHS trusts and one SHA. By June 2005 one NHS trust had been franchised to an independent sector provider.

Structure

In mid-2004, 249 independent sector hospitals, in the voluntary sector as well as the private sector, were registered to take inpatients and day-cases, with some 9,176 acute (or secondary care) medical and surgical beds.[71] ‡ Besides profit-making companies the 'private' sector also includes organisations such as Nuffield Hospitals Trust and BUPA, which are described as 'provident funds'; they make

---

* NHS standards refer to those assessed by the Healthcare Commission (see Chapter 6, pages 110–11); the NHS tariff refers to the standard price paid to all providers of NHS care for a given procedure (see Chapter 5 pages 97–8).

† In mid-2005 the independent sector providers on the register were Bupa, BMI, the Swedish owned Capio, Interhealth Canada, Hospitalia Active Health (from Germany), Serco (the British owned facilities management company), Secta Group and the consultancy firm Quo Health.

‡ There were also 175 private and voluntary hospitals providing psychiatric inpatient services (including substance misuse treatment) and/or rehabilitation services, and 109 private pathology laboratories. Source: Laing and Buisson (2004), *Laing's Healthcare Market Review, 2004–2005,* London, pp. 188 and 114.

profits, but re-invest them in services and salaries rather than distributing them to shareholders. In mid-2003, however, 68 per cent of hospitals, beds and revenue in the independent sector as a whole were owned by for-profit providers.[72] With ongoing mergers and acquisitions the sector is currently dominated by five hospital providers, owning some 78 per cent of hospital beds. Three of these are UK-based, the others being UK subsidiaries of Swedish- and US-based companies.[73] The US and other trans-national hospital groups operating in the UK generate a particularly high level of revenue per bed.[74]

NHS trusts have also increased their own provision of private facilities and services. For example in 2001 University College London Hospitals NHS Trust acquired a private hospital providing cardio-thoracic services, while in 2002 the Hammersmith Hospital acquired the Masonic Stamford Hospital on a 15-year lease.

Although the DH considers the use of independent sector staff a way to help overcome NHS staff shortages, most of the work undertaken by the independent sector uses nursing and medical staff trained in, and for the most part still employed by, the NHS. The latest data identify almost 9,000 qualified nursing or mid-wifery staff employed by independent sector hospitals or clinics,[75] most of whom were trained in the NHS. Similarly in 1999 there were 16,000 NHS consultants in England who spent at least part of their time practising in the private sector.[76]

Joint ventures

Partnerships between NHS bodies and the private sector are an integral part of the government's plan to modernise the NHS. For the purpose of building new hospitals NHS trusts have had this ability since the 1990s, through the Private Finance Initiative or PFI discussed more fully in Chapter 5 (pages 90–1). The 2001 Health and Social Care Act extended these powers to SHAs and PCTs, enabling them to participate in public–private partnerships to develop primary care premises through the Local Improvement Finance Trust (LIFT) initiative (again discussed more fully in Chapter 5, pages 94–5).

The 2001 Health and Social Care Act also enabled NHS bodies to form partnerships or 'joint ventures' with private companies for the purpose of generating income. Approval is required from the Secretary of State for Health, who may also provide assets, loans and financial guarantees. Thus, NHS trusts, PCTs and care trusts may form partnerships with companies for the purpose of generating income with capital provided by the NHS. Such companies may supply healthcare goods or services, or exploit intellectual property, for example by marketing technological advances and findings from research studies. For FTs such ventures are not limited to healthcare activities.

At the national level the DH and the private sector firm Xansa have formed a joint venture company called NHS Shared Business Services Limited. This provides 'back office work' such as payment of invoices, VAT returns, debt collection and bank account reconciliation from two service centres in Leeds and Bristol. At the local level some NHS trusts have undertaken joint ventures with independent sector hospitals: for example the General Healthcare Group operates six 'partnership projects' on NHS sites.[77] In this model the private hospital takes on the development costs, pays rent, purchases services such as pathology from the NHS trust, and may often 'sell' clinical services to the NHS trust. In another example, the University Hospitals Coventry and Warwickshire NHS Trust has formed a partnership with BMI healthcare for the joint management of a new NHS private patient unit.

Treatment overseas

Under EU legislation NHS patients are entitled to seek treatment in other European Union member states at NHS expense. The use of overseas medical providers has also been recognised by the DH as a means of accessing extra capacity, in order to help NHS trusts and PCTs experiencing capacity shortfalls to reduce waiting lists for elective procedures in specialties such as orthopaedics, ophthalmology and cardiology.

Since 2002 PCTs have been able to offer overseas treatment to patients who have been waiting relatively long periods for elective treatment and who are clinically fit to travel. Following a 'referral' from an NHS trust, PCTs commission procedures from hospital providers in Northern Europe, at costs comparable with those for patients treated in the private sector in England. By March 2004 nearly 750 people had been treated in Europe through these arrangements in France, Germany and Belgium, predominantly for orthopaedic and cardiac procedures.[78]

The procurement process is undertaken on behalf of PCTs by a 'lead' commissioner, currently either Kent and Medway SHA or Guy's and St Thomas's hospital in London. The lead commissioner identifies European hospital providers, negotiates prices, organises patients' travel and monitors the quality of services provided, examining accreditation systems, infection control processes, and post-operative infection and complication rates, and ensuring that the Healthcare Commission (see Chapter 6, pages 116–17) has contractual visiting rights at the overseas hospitals in question. The lead commissioner also holds the contract with the European hospital; PCTs take out 'service level agreements' (NHS-type contracts) with the lead commissioner rather than with the overseas healthcare provider itself.

The DH has stated that 'the law on the commissioner's liability for clinical issues is not wholly clear'.[79] But patients treated abroad retain the right to sue the NHS in the English courts for the quality of care they receive; prime liability remains with the 'referring' NHS trust.

Public health

Public health is concerned with health of the population as opposed to the individual. This is a broad remit, encompassing issues ranging from health promotion activities such as reducing smoking rates, through a wide range of health protection activities such as communicable disease control and protecting against the effects of bio-terrorism, to the reduction of inequalities in health. The importance of the public health agenda has been recognised by the DH, which has stated its intention to adopt a more holistic approach, developing the NHS 'into a health service rather than one that focuses primarily on sickness'.[80] A number of core functions have been described for the public health system in England (Box 4.1), which includes not only the NHS organisations described below but also bodies such as local authorities and voluntary organisations.

The Department of Health

At the DH a parliamentary under-secretary of state for public health is responsible for policies relating to preventative services, communicable diseases and sexual health, health inequalities, drugs, tobacco and alcohol, sustainable development, cancer, coronary heart disease, tobacco policy, communicable diseases and their control, immunisation, health inequalities, drug and alcohol misuse, sexual health issues and food safety. He or she is advised by the the chief medical officer (CMO), whose remit also includes: developing and implementing policies to protect the health of the public, such as the 2004 'action plan' detailing activities to be undertaken by NHS and other organisations to help control the rise of tuberculosis; promoting and taking action to improve the health of the population and reduce inequalities, such as publishing a 2004 white paper outlining health promotion activities aimed at reducing smoking and obesity rates; and leading initiatives to enhance the quality and safety of services within the NHS, such as proposals to prevent, identify and deal with poorly-performing doctors. The CMO also sits on the DH's board of directors, and leads the Health and Social Care

---

Box 4.1   Core functions of the public health system in England

- Health surveillance, monitoring and analysis
- Investigation of disease outbreaks, epidemics, and risks to health
- Health promotion and disease prevention programmes
- Enabling and empowering communities and citizens to promote health and reduce inequalities
- Creating and sustaining cross-governmental and inter-sectoral partnerships to improve health and reduce inequalities
- Ensuring compliance with regulations and laws to promote and protect health
- Developing and maintaining the public health workforce
- Ensuring that NHS services improve health, prevent disease and reduce inequalities
- Research, development, evaluation and innovation

Source: Department of Health website.

Standards and Quality Group within whose remit the public health function falls (see Chapter 2, page 15).

The public health responsibility of the DH is supported by nine regional directors of public health, who are accountable to the CMO. To make possible greater integration between their work and that of non-NHS organisations, since April 2002 they have been located within the government offices of the regions. Their role is to develop and 'mentor' the public health functions within their regions, and to address public health issues and health inequalities at the regional level.

SHAs, PCTs, and public health networks

In 2001 a DH paper entitled *Shifting the Balance of Power* outlined a restructuring of the delivery system of the NHS, including arrangements intended to strengthen the public health function at the regional, and particularly at the local, level. Every SHA is now required to appoint a senior public health doctor or medical director to oversee and co-ordinate the public health function in all the PCTs in the SHA's area. Every PCT should have a director of public health (DPH) at board level. DPHs lead on public health issues, supporting a diverse range of public health staff such as consultants and specialists in public health medicine*, health visitors,† consultants in communicable disease control, infection control nurses, information analysts, health promotion workers and community outreach workers.

Within PCTs the public health function is about improving the health and well-being of the local population and reducing inequalities in health. This involves identifying the local population's health and healthcare needs, using epidemiological and health service data, consulting with organisations and local communities, and then providing services to meet the needs identified. These services include preventative and health promotion activities such as screening, immunisation and smoking cessation services, helping to plan the provision of clinical and other services to meet the local population's healthcare needs, and helping managers evaluate and maximise the effectiveness of services. The public health function is also about tackling inequalities in health and the wider determinants of ill-health, such as poverty, poor housing and poor education. To address these issues public health practitioners work in partnership with other organisations such as local authorities and private, business, community and voluntary organisations, helping them deliver local 'neighbourhood renewal

---

* These are practitioners in public health from a non-medical background but who have achieved similar standards in the practice of public health to those of medically trained practitioners and have been awarded a status equivalent to that of consultant by the Faculty of Public Health.

† Health visitors are responsible for the health of babies and young children in the community. They play an important public health role, especially through promoting healthy lifestyles within families and encouraging the uptake of vaccines and immunisation.

strategies' and other initiatives such as 'healthy eating' in schools, and schemes to increase people's levels of physical activity.

The public health function encompasses a broad spectrum of work areas. Recognising that the necessary expertise could not be provided in all 303 PCTs in England, *Shifting the Balance of Power* also led to the introduction of public health networks. These are linked groups of public health professionals with a common agenda to promote health improvement and reduce inequalities, who work in a co-ordinated manner across organisational boundaries. They include informal networks, such as e-mail groups concerned with particular topics, as well as formal 'managed networks' for the provision of specific services.

Managed networks are intended to facilitate the pooling of skills and expertise and to prevent the professional isolation which can occur in organisations with small numbers of public health staff serving relatively small populations, such as PCTs. They are also intended to make it possible to co-ordinate specialist public health work, facilitating the planning of public health interventions at local and regional level. They can operate within and between PCTs, their structures reflecting local needs and organisational issues. Their members may include public health specialists, public health practitioners such as health visitors, and people from non-NHS organisations such as academic departments and local authorities.

Public health observatories

Public health observatories (PHOs) were established in February 2000 following the 1999 white paper *Saving Lives: Our Healthier Nation*. There are now nine observatories across England, aligned with regional government office boundaries plus others in Wales and Northern Ireland.* They monitor regional trends in health and health care and help evaluate the progress of local agencies in improving health by drawing together information from different sources such as the Office for National Statistics, local authorities, the NHS, and the police. They also provide a regional hospital episode statistics (HES) data service, producing comparative analyses of hospital admissions at regional level. Working through the Association of Public Health Observatories they constitute a national network of public health knowledge, information and surveillance, producing summary reports of public health indicators[†] across the English regions; undertaking 'lead' work, such as the London Health Observatory's development of a 'basket' of indicators for use at

---

*   The English observatories are in London, Mansfield (the East Midlands), Stockton-on-Tees (the North East), Liverpool (the North West), Oxford (the South East), Bristol (the South West), Cambridge (Eastern Region), Birmingham (the West Midlands) and York (Yorkshire and Humber).

†   These include population health status indicators such as life expectancy, priority public health interventions such as screening and immunisation rates, effectiveness in partnerships such as reduction in teenage pregnancy rates, wider determinants of health and risk factors such as smoking rates, and public health capacity, such as the number of public health trainees per million population.

local level to monitor inequalities in health and its determinants; and collaborating with other organisations, for example the South East PHO's collaboration with the British Heart Foundation to produce a series of national analyses of coronary heart disease data.

PHOs are centrally funded by the DH, although this income can be supplemented by income generated by work undertaken for other organisations. Staffed mainly by public health specialists and information analysts, PHOs vary in size, but even the London Health Observatory, for example, covers a population of seven million people with just 19 staff.[79] As NHS bodies PHOs are overseen by boards, although unlike NHS trusts and PCTs their members are drawn purely from key partner organisations (such as SHAs, PCTs, local authorities or academic institutions) and there is no requirement for 'lay' or 'public' membership. In conjunction with the regional Director of Public Health the board of each PHO oversees its work, as well as advising on priorities for future work. Each board is also collectively accountable to a national (England-wide) governing board which includes many DH representatives and is chaired by the CMO.

The National Institute for Health and Clinical Excellence

Responsibility for identifying the evidence base for public health and health promotion interventions now lies with the National Institute for Health and Clinical Excellence (NICE), described more fully in Chapters 2 and 6 (pages 28–9, and 113–14).

The public health role of NICE is to gather evidence on the effectiveness of interventions to improve population health and reduce health inequalities. This is undertaken by its Centre for Public Health Excellence, through a series of work programmes intended to build on the work of its forerunner, the Health Development Agency. This includes work such as the publication of briefings and reviews of evidence relating to health promotion activities, for example on interventions to promote healthy eating or tackle alcohol misuse; the maintenance of a number of websites and electronic databases providing access to such evidence; and publishing guidance on best practice to help get the evidence used in practice.

The Health Protection Agency

The Health Protection Agency (HPA) was first proposed in 2002, in a report by the Chief Medical Officer, entitled *Getting Ahead of the Curve*. With increased numbers of people living with HIV/AIDS infection, and the high-profile crisis of BSE, the report recognised the persistence of the threat of infectious diseases, due both to the re-emergence of diseases such as tuberculosis and the possibility of deliberately-released disease organisms in acts of bio-terrorism. It recommended the establishment of a new agency to co-ordinate the functions of infection control and health protection.

The HPA was first established in April 2003 as a special health authority covering England and Wales, but in April 2005 it was re-established as a UK-wide non-departmental public body (see Chapter 2, page 30). Through the merger of a number of existing organisations and functions it has become responsible for a wide range of health protection functions relating to biological, chemical and radiological hazards, and for emergency planning. It has subsumed the Centres for Communicable Disease Control and the Public Health Laboratory Service; the National Poisons Information Centre; and the National Focus for Chemical Incidents and its regional service provider units, which supported the management of chemical incidents. It has also incorporated the work of Consultants in Communicable Disease Control and regional emergency planning advisers, and in 2005 also subsumed the National Radiological Protection Board. By April 2006 it will also have taken over the functions of the National Institute for Biological Standards and Control, which standardises and controls the biological materials used in medicines.

With a budget of £221.8 million in 2004–5 the HPA had a total of over 3,000 staff,[81] including specialists in communicable disease control, infection control nurses, public health specialists, microbiologists, toxicologists, laboratory scientists and technicians, epidemiologists, information specialists, and emergency planning advisers. As in other NHS organisations the work and strategic direction of the HPA is overseen by a board who are collectively accountable for its performance and use of public funds. The board, appointed by the NHS Appointments Commission, consists of between 10 and 15 members drawn from the HPA and other organisations, comprising a range of experience reflecting the functions of the HPA. They are accountable to the Secretary of State for Health, and like other NHS organisations are required to produce an annual report and undergo an annual financial audit from an auditor appointed by the Audit Commission.

The role of the HPA is to prevent and control the spread of infectious diseases, reduce the adverse effects of chemical hazards, poisons and radiation, and prepare for potential or emerging threats to health (such as the international outbreak of sudden acute respiratory syndrome or SARS in 2003). It also has an important role in research and development, and in education and training matters relating to health protection. It provides advice and support services to the government, health professionals and the public through four operational 'divisions', in addition to a business division which provides corporate and other support functions for the organisation as a whole. The four operational divisions are:

The centre for infections

The centre for infections undertakes monitoring and surveillance of infectious diseases and provides a national reference microbiology service. The latter has facilities for the identification of rare pathogens such as diphtheria, provides national and international laboratory quality assurance schemes, and deploys sophisticated techniques such as microbial strain characterisation. These services are provided through a network of reference laboratories, including regional and hospital laboratories as well as national facilities such as those at Porton Down and Colindale.

The centre for radiation, environmental and chemical hazards

This division took over the functions of the National Radiological Protection Board, providing information and advice to the Government and agencies responsible for protecting the public from radiation hazards, including hazard control procedures as well as emergency planning for radiation incidents. It also provides environmental monitoring as well as advice and support for chemical incidents, such as decontamination, evacuation, antidotes and medical treatment, as well as a national programme for the surveillance of chemical hazards. It also provides a National Poisons Information Service, with six poisons information centres which provide information for healthcare professionals on the management of patients who may have been poisoned.

The emergency response division

This division is responsible for improving the preparedness of the NHS and other agencies to respond to major incidents, such as outbreaks of disease, chemical spills, or the deliberate release of harmful substances. This work includes providing specialist advice on both the planning for, and the operational response to, such incidents, providing training and information for staff and running exercises to test the emergency responses of local organisations.

The local and regional services division

The fourth division is the largest in the HPA. Its role is to coordinate services at the local and regional level, acting as a source of specialist advice and operational support for local NHS organisations, local authorities and other agencies. It operates through nine regional offices corresponding to the government offices of the region (the same as those of the public health observatories described on pages 74–5). Each regional team provides epidemiology, microbiology, and emergency planning functions; its role is to help the regional director of public health to manage the responses to major incidents and to co-ordinate the activities of the local health protection units (HPUs) within its area.

There are 39 HPUs across England, with boundaries generally co-terminous with county or police boundaries. Staffed by consultants, nurses and other personnel with specialist health protection skills, they work in collaboration with PCTs, NHS trusts and local authorities to deliver health protection functions at the local level. This includes disease surveillance and alert systems and the investigation and management of health protection incidents, such as chemical hazards and infectious disease outbreaks.

5 Funding and resources

UK expenditure on healthcare has always been comparatively low, but since the year 2000 a major increase in expenditure on the NHS has been a key policy aim of the Labour government. For the UK as a whole government spending on the NHS rose from 5.4 per cent of GDP* in 1997[1] to 7.1 per cent in 2005–6. It will rise further, to 7.8 per cent of GDP, by 2007–8 (Table 5.1).

Government funding of the NHS accounts for 82 per cent of all expenditure on healthcare; the other 18 per cent is accounted for by private medical insurance (both company and personal schemes), and by self-paying private patients.[2] The increases in government spending mean that total expenditure on healthcare, (i.e. including both government and private expenditure) will reach 9.2 per cent of GDP by 2007–8. This will still be less than in comparable countries such as France, Germany and the United States, which in 2003 were already spending 10, 11.5 and 15 per cent of their GDP respectively on health care (Table 5.2).

Government expenditure on the NHS is funded mainly from general taxation, accounting for 74 per cent of its funding in 2005–6. This was supplemented by national insurance contributions (20 per cent of the total), plus a small contribution from charges (e.g. for prescriptions and dentistry) and from the proceeds of land

---

* The Gross Domestic Product is a measure of the total economic production of a country or area over a specified period, usually a year.

Table 5.1 Planned expenditure on healthcare in the UK, as a percentage of gross domestic product (GDP), 2005–6 to 2007–8

	% of GDP	
	2005–6	*2007–8*
Government expenditure	7.1	7.8
Private expenditure	1.4	1.4
Total UK expenditure	8.6	9.2

Source: HM Treasury (2004) government spending review, Chapter 8.

Table 5.2 Expenditure on healthcare as a percentage of gross domestic product (GDP), by country

Country	Expenditure (% of GDP)
UK: planned expenditure for 2007–8[1]	9.2
Actual expenditure for 2003[2]	
France	10
Germany	11.5
United States	15

Notes
1 HM Treasury, 2004 spending review, Chapter 8.
2 Organisation for Economic Co-operation and Development, Health data 2005.

sales and income-generation schemes.[3] All this expenditure is said to be 'cash-limited': the total is determined in advance by the Treasury in consultation with the Department of Health (DH), which determines how to allocate the funds. Since 1998 these decisions have been made in the context of a three-yearly public spending 'round', taking place within comprehensive spending reviews of total government expenditure.

The allocation of resources for the NHS in England*

Government expenditure on the NHS in England equalled £76 billion in 2005–6, and will rise to £92 billion by 2007–8.[2] The DH allocates these resources to the NHS according to the 'supply estimates' approved by the Treasury. *Revenue allocations* cover running costs such as staff salaries and wages and the purchase of goods and services, including drugs and fuel. *Capital allocations* are for purchasing and maintaining assets which provide benefits for more than a year, such as land, buildings and medical equipment.

Revenue allocation

In 2005–6 revenue allocations accounted for £72.2 billion, 95 per cent of the total NHS allocation. A relatively small portion of this (£3 billion) is allocated to cover the DH's administrative costs and so-called 'central health and miscellaneous services', such as the various special agencies described in Chapter 2 (pages 20–34); research and development funds; and the medical costs of UK nationals treated in European Union member states. Ninety-eight per cent of revenue allocations, however, are for the provision of hospital, community and family health services – £70.6 billion in 2005–6.[4] In the past expenditure on hospital

*   The relevant data are not reported for the UK as a whole. Unless otherwise indicated the data in the rest of this chapter are for England only.

services has always accounted for over 50 per cent of the allocations for hospital, community and family health service allocations (see Figure 5.1); this percentage should decline, however, as new initiatives take effect to shift service provision to community settings.

Funding streams for the allocation of revenue for hospital, community and family health services

Revenue for hospital, community and family health services is allocated through different funding streams (Figure 5.2): 'direct' or 'unified' allocations to primary care trusts (PCTs), 'central budgets', non-discretionary funding streams (to reimburse ophthalmic and pharmaceutical practitioners), and allocations to PCTs for NHS dental services.

DIRECT ALLOCATIONS TO PCTS

Most revenue for hospital, community and family health services is allocated directly to PCTs as 'unified allocations'. PCTs use these funds to commission hospital, community and primary care medical services for their local populations from NHS trusts, foundation trusts, treatment centres, independent providers, and GP practices. SHAs' running costs are also met out of their local PCTs' allocations. In 2005–6, PCTs received £58.9 billion as direct or 'unified' allocations, equivalent to 78 per cent of total government expenditure on the NHS.[4] Since 2003 these allocations have been made in advance on a three-yearly basis, to enable PCTs to plan ahead.

PCTs' 'unified' allocations are supplemented by revenue allocated to them from the DH's central budgets to pay for 'centrally funded initiatives and services', such

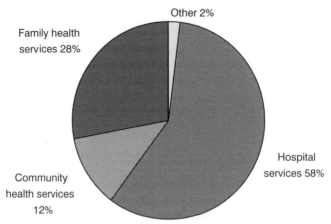

Figure 5.1   How expenditure is divided between hospital and other health services, 2002–3
House of Commons Health committee, *Public Expenditure on Health and Personal Social Services*; London 2005.

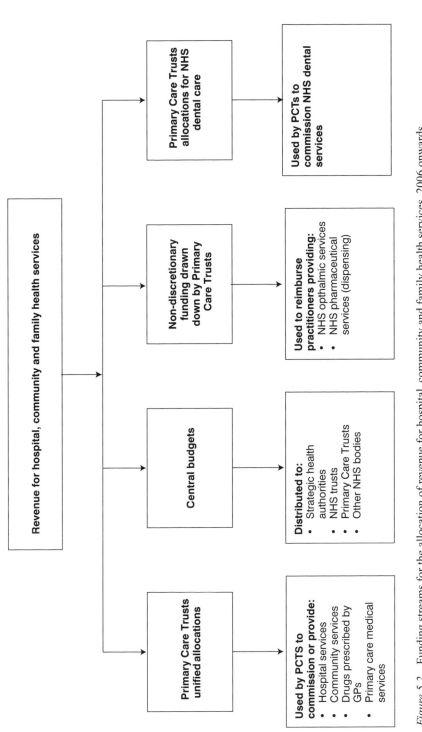

Revenue for hospital, community and family health services

Primary Care Trusts unified allocations

Used by PCTS to commission or provide:
- Hospital services
- Community services
- Drugs prescribed by GPs
- Primary care medical services

Central budgets

Distributed to:
- Strategic health authorities
- NHS trusts
- Primary Care Trusts
- Other NHS bodies

Non-discretionary funding drawn down by Primary Care Trusts

Used to reimburse practitioners providing:
- NHS opthalmic services
- NHS pharmaceutical services (dispensing)

Primary Care Trusts allocations for NHS dental care

Used by PCTs to commission NHS dental services

Figure 5.2   Funding streams for the allocation of revenue for hospital, community and family health services, 2006 onwards

as smoking cessation services and electronic hospital appointment booking systems. These allocations came to £3 billion in 2005–6, increasing PCTs' share of total NHS expenditure to 81 per cent.[4] These two sources of revenue form a 'resource limit' for each PCT, within which they must contain their overall expenditure. They are, however, free to determine the relative shares of the total to be spent on each of the various elements of hospital, community and family health services, such as particular hospital services, community health services, drugs prescribed by GPs, and, from April 2006 onwards, primary care medical services provided by GPs. The only exceptions are certain elements of primary care; some GP practice payments are ring-fenced,* and there is also a 'floor 'level' of expenditure on so-called 'enhanced services'† (see Chapter 4, page 51) on which PCTs are required to spend a minimum amount (£700 million for England in 2005–6).[5]

CENTRAL BUDGETS

As mentioned above, the DH allocates some funding for centrally-determined specific purposes, distributing it to SHAs, NHS trusts and PCTs, as well as to specialised agencies. This funding covers items such as the education and training of NHS staff, research and development support, and the work of the NHS Litigation Authority (see Chapter 2, pages 25–7). It is also used to pay for 'centrally funded initiatives and services', such as meeting the waiting-time targets in the NHS Plan through the implementation of electronic booking systems for hospital appointments and admissions. In 2005–6 the money in these central budgets totalled £11.7 billion, or 16 per cent of all DH revenue allocations.[4]

NON-DISCRETIONARY FUNDING STREAMS

'Non-discretionary' funding is held by the DH and 'drawn down' by PCTs to reimburse practitioners for providing NHS ophthalmic and pharmaceutical (dispensing) services. Theoretically there is no upper limit to the money which can be claimed through these funding streams, but the schedule of reimbursement is set on the basis of expected activity in order to maintain expenditure within budgetary constraints. In 2003–4 expenditure was £304 million on NHS ophthalmic services and £918 million on NHS pharmaceutical (dispensing) services.[6]

FUNDING FOR NHS DENTAL SERVICES

NHS dental services have traditionally been funded in a manner similar to NHS pharmaceutical and ophthalmic services: money was 'drawn down' from the DH

---

*   Under the general medical services (GMS) contract introduced in 2004 the 'global sum' which practices receive to cover running costs is 'ring-fenced', meaning that it must all be paid directly to them.

†   'Enhanced services' are more specialised services delivered within primary care, such as minor surgery, or primary care for patients with histories of violent behaviour.

by the NHS Business Services Authority (described in Chapter 2, page 25) to reimburse practitioners for providing NHS dental services. In April 2006, however, PCTs will assume responsibility for commissioning NHS dental services and will receive specific revenue allocations for this purpose, broadly based on the historical level of expenditure on NHS dental services, which was expected to be £1.6 billion for England in 2005–6.[7] At the time of writing it is undecided whether this will be allocated separately or included within the unified allocations given to PCTs; the matter is to be reviewed approximately three years after the commissioning of dental services by PCTs has been introduced.

The distribution of direct or unified allocations to PCTs

As already mentioned, most PCT revenue consists of 'direct' or 'unified' allocations to pay for hospital, community and family health services. Certain elements of these allocations are distributed to PCTs using allocation formulae, the aim of which is to distribute revenue in such a way as to secure equal opportunity of access to health care for people of equal need. Different formulae are used for different services, namely for the hospital and community health services, services for people with HIV/AIDS, the costs of prescribed drugs, and certain elements of primary care. Revenue for the remaining elements of primary care, such as funding for practices which provide services under PMS arrangements (see Chapter 4, page 52), or quality payments to 'reward' good practice, is distributed either according to historical arrangements or through a 'quality and outcomes' framework. The sum of all these elements, each of which is described below, contributes a PCTs 'direct' or 'unified' allocation.

REVENUE ALLOCATION FORMULAE: HOSPITAL AND COMMUNITY HEALTH SERVICES AND ELEMENTS OF PRIMARY CARE

The allocation formulae used to distribute revenue according to local needs for all these various services are shown in Figure 5.3. These formulae, however, do not at present determine PCTs' actual allocations. Their actual allocations, known as 'recurrent baselines', are inherited from an earlier system of allocation.* They are in fact the previous year's allocations, plus any adjustments made over the current financial year. The allocation formulae shown in Figure 5.3 yield a different result, known as the 'fair share' or 'target allocation' for each PCT. Their actual

---

* Following the work of the Resource Allocation Working Party (RAWP) in the 1970s, and subsequent reviews by the Advisory Committee on Resource Allocation (ACRA), revenue for the hospital and community health services began to be distributed on the basis of 'weighted capitation'. Resident population size was adjusted by various proxy measures of the need for services, and the costs of providing services, in different areas. Revenue for primary care services was distributed to individual GPs on the basis of their list size or 'capitation', supplemented by a complicated system of fees and allowances detailed in the DH's 'red book' for items such as infrastructure, and for achieving specific targets such as immunisation rates.

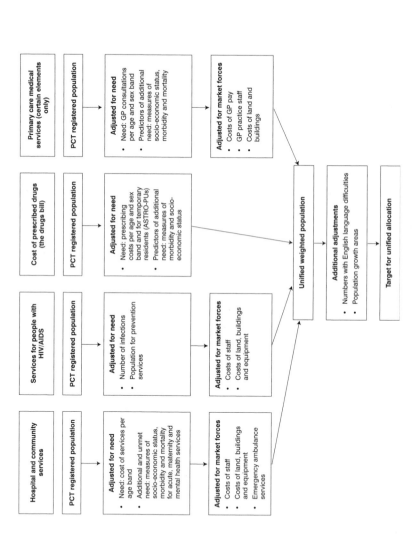

Figure 5.3 How the target allocation of resources for hospital and other health services is determined

allocations, or 'recurrent baselines', are brought nearer to the target allocations through the distribution of any *increased* spending, at a speed determined by ministers and known as the 'pace of change'. PCTs in more deprived areas – so-called 'spearhead PCTs', which are the furthest from their target allocations – receive the greatest increases. The aim is that all PCTs should reach their target allocations by 2010.

The allocation formulae are known as 'weighted capitation' formulae. This means that they are based on population numbers, or 'capitation', weighted for measures of healthcare need such as morbidity and mortality rates and the level of use of services. They are also adjusted for 'market forces' – unavoidable differences in the costs of providing services in different areas. A number of new policy initiatives may, however, make these adjustments redundant. With 'patient choice' (see Chapter 4, page 62, and below, pages 98–9) whereby patients will be able to choose any national provider, the use of services will no longer be an accurate reflection of local need.

It is the patients registered with the GP practices within a PCT, rather than geographically-defined resident populations, who form the 'capitation' basis for the formulae. These numbers are determined from information collected on the PCTs' 'Exeter' software systems, extracted and held nationally and known as the 'attribution data set'. These figures are then 'reconciled with', or scaled back to, the resident populations, as given by the national census, to ensure that PCT populations add up to the national population of England, and that imperfections in the records of patients on the practice lists in different parts of the country do not affect the allocation of revenue.[*]

The revenue allocation formulae are used to distribute resources for those elements of primary care services that are covered by GMS arrangements (see Chapter 4, page 51). These include both 'essential' and 'additional' services, for which GP practices receive a payment known as the 'global sum'. Calculated quarterly and paid monthly, the 'global sum' is a 'ring-fenced' allocation, distributed to each GP practice – PCTs act only as intermediaries for its distribution. 'Global sum' allocations for England totalled £1.9 billion in 2005–6;[8] an 'average' GP practice, with three whole-time-equivalent GP principals and a list of 5,500 patients, received £54 per patient or £305,000 per annum.[9] Practices opting out of providing 'additional' or out-of-hours services have their global sum reduced according to a national tariff, adjusted by the practice's weighted population; an 'average' GP practice choosing not to provide out-of-hours services, for example, has its global sum reduced by 6 per cent.[10]

The revenue allocation formulae also allocate revenue according to the need for GP infrastructure (information technology and existing premises), and the need for 'enhanced' services (such as minor surgery, etc. – see Chapter 4, page 51). In 2005–6 PCTs received a total of £546 million for these purposes.[8]

---

[*] This is intended to ensure that the whole population of England is covered by the NHS, in contrast to other register-based systems, such as the one used in the United States, where people not registered with a healthcare organisation have no healthcare cover.

FUNDING FOR PMS PRACTICES

When the new funding arrangements for primary care were introduced in 2004, just over 40 per cent of GPs were working under PMS arrangements (see Chapter 4, page 52).[11] PCTs receive a separate revenue allocation to enable them to honour existing PMS commitments. Amounting to £1.9 billion in 2005–6,[8] this figure was arrived at by 'uplifting' the previous year's allocations for PMS practices to cover the effects of price inflation. These allocations represent the sum of all the practice allocations negotiated locally between PCTs and individual practices. Remuneration was set at the level of past years in order to protect practices' levels of income. New PMS schemes, however, and new investments in existing PMS schemes, are to be paid for by identifying funds that can be transferred from the other elements of PCTs' primary care medical services allocations.

QUALITY PAYMENTS TO GP PRACTICES: THE 'QUALITY AND OUTCOMES FRAMEWORK'

PCTs are also allocated revenue to pay to GP practices according to the 'quality' of services they provide – a system of financial incentives intended to reward good practice through voluntary participation in an annual quality improvement cycle known as the 'quality and outcomes framework'. The framework contains 146 indicators organised within four domains; a clinical domain, with indicators such as keeping a coronary heart disease register or providing smoking cessation advice;* an organisational domain, with indicators such as recording patient measurements and keeping up-to-date patient summaries; an 'additional services' domain, with indicators relating to the provision of services such as cervical screening; and a 'patient experience' domain, with indicators such as the length of consultations and whether practices survey patient experience.

Revenue is allocated to PCTs on the basis of the expected performance of the GP practices in their area, adjusted for practices' list sizes and for disease prevalence. The sum involved amounted to £1 billion for England in 2005–6.[12] PCTs distribute these funds to GP practices on a 'points' system. Through discussion with their PCT, practices are awarded points both for aspiring to achieve indicators of their choice, and for subsequently achieving them. Each point has a monetary value, worth £120 to a practice in 2005–6.[13] For indicators in the clinical domain the figures are adjusted for the disease prevalence within the practice, and for indicators in the 'additional services' domain they are adjusted for the size of the practice's target population relative to the national average. Payments for the four domains are then added together and adjusted for the practice's list size relative to the national average. If practices in general perform better than expected it will obviously lead to more money being paid out than was budgeted for; in 2004–5 the expected achievement of 85 per cent was in fact exceeded by

---

* Clinical indicators are organised by disease category. They were selected from conditions where responsibility for ongoing patient management lies principally within primary care; where there is good evidence that improved primary care can lead to health benefits; and where the disease area is a priority.

practices in England. The DH intend, however, that the framework should lead to better chronic disease management, which should improve health outcomes and reduce avoidable hospital attendances, and so reduce overall costs.[14]

Other revenue

A relatively small amount of PCTs' revenue is allocated through an assortment of other funding streams. For example in 2006–7 and 2007–8 PCTs in England will receive allocations totalling £211 million and £131 million to fund the implementation of the government's 2004 white paper on public health, *Choosing Health*, targeted at PCTs serving relatively deprived areas.[15] These funds are intended to be used not only for improvements in primary care but also for public health initiatives such as school nurses and health trainers who will work with children to tackle obesity, and improved services for sexually-transmitted diseases.

Other (non-DH) sources of funding for PCTs

In addition to funding from the DH, recent legislation has given PCTs access to a number of new funding streams. The 1999 Health Act enabled them to pool specific budgets with those of local authorities, for example when securing services for the elderly or for people with learning disabilities. This freedom was extended under the 2001 Health and Social Care Act to allow PCTs to form Care Trusts (see Chapter 4, pages 44–6), which are voluntary partnerships between PCTs and local authorities. This gives PCTs access to local authority funding, which includes both government revenue and revenue from means-tested user charges for services (since local authority social services are charged for). By 2004 some 130 schemes using one or more of these flexibilities were known to be in place.[16]

Under the 1988 Health and Medicines Act PCTs can also generate additional income to fund the delivery of NHS services. Provided such activities do not disadvantage NHS patients, PCTs can acquire, produce and market goods and services, and exploit marketable service innovations and intellectual property rights. The 2001 Health and Social Care Act also allowed them to form 'spin-off' (or 'spin-out') companies either alone or in partnership with the private sector, with the purpose of generating income from activities such as running nursing homes or selling clinical services (for example pathology services carried out on behalf of a private hospital).

Capital allocation

Capital allocations are made to NHS bodies to fund the purchase and replacement of NHS assets – items which provide benefits for more than one year, such as land, buildings and medical equipment. Different systems are used to allocate capital for the hospital and community health services, and for primary care, but in both cases capital expenditure is increasingly being supplemented from the revenue allocations of NHS bodies. This arises from the requirement that NHS bodies must pay 'capital charges' – an annual 'interest' payment to the Treasury for the use of their capital assets, described below (page 100) – out of their revenue funding streams. The increasing use of private funding for NHS capital investments is also paid for out of the revenue allocations of NHS bodies.

Capital allocation for the hospital and community health services

In 2000 the total NHS 'estate' – predominantly the land, buildings and equipment used for the provision of hospital and community health services – was valued at approximately £23 billion.[17] * Most of these assets are owned by NHS trusts, but with an associated debt to the Treasury which must be repaid if the assets are sold. PCTs also own their own premises, and may also own health centres or community sites from which they provide community health services.

Individual NHS trusts and PCTs are responsible for purchasing, maintaining and improving their own assets, using a variety of funding mechanisms. They receive dedicated capital allocations from the DH, which they can supplement with operating surpluses known as 'internally generated resources', and with receipts from property and land sales. But private finance, in the form of the Private Finance Initiative or PFI, has now become the major source of funding for new capital investment in the NHS. Foundation trusts operate under different capital funding arrangements and are considered separately.

DEDICATED CAPITAL ALLOCATIONS

As with revenue allocations, capital allocations are made for three-year periods; NHS organisations receive only one year's capital funding at a time, but are told their allocations for three-year periods to facilitate the planning of services and investments. New allocation formulae were introduced in 2003 in an attempt to distribute funds in relation to the need for capital investment. This distribution takes place through four separate funding streams: operational capital, strategic capital, the access fund, and centrally-held programme capital. Taken together they amounted to some £4 billion in 2005–6. [18]

1) OPERATIONAL CAPITAL   Operational capital is allocated for the maintenance of minor assets, such as the replacement of equipment. Just over £1 billion was allocated for this purpose in 2005–6, distributed directly to NHS trusts (and to a lesser extent to PCTs, which own comparatively few assets). It is distributed using

---

*   This figure excludes most GP premises, which are in private ownership, as explained on page 92.

an allocation formula based on the depreciation of organisations' assets. Ninety-two per cent of the available funds are distributed according to each organisation's share of the total national depreciation cost of NHS assets, while the remaining 8 per cent is targeted at organisations with highly depreciated (i.e. badly run-down) assets. As with revenue allocations, this formula does not determine an organisation's actual allocation, but yields a 'target' allocation. Ministers decide the 'pace of change', i.e. how quickly organisations are moved from their historical allocations to their target allocations, although during the post-2000 increase in government funding for the NHS all organisations are currently receiving at least 7 per cent more operational capital each year.

2) STRATEGIC CAPITAL   Strategic capital allocations pay for major investments, such as new buildings and major refurbishments. They are distributed to SHAs on the basis of weighted capitation, using the same formula as is used to allocate revenue to PCTs for hospital and community health services (see Figure 5.3 above). This is further adjusted to account for the flow of patients across the geographic boundaries of PCTs, to ensure that the allocations go to the areas where patients are actually being treated. In 2005–6, £866 million was distributed between the 28 SHAs, in allocations ranging from £17 million to £46 million.[18]

SHAs are responsible for distributing the allocations within their areas, allocating resources in order to meet national priorities such as improving access and implementing the national programme for information technology. They are able to approve bids from NHS organisations (known as 'business cases') up to a value of £25 million without seeking approval from the DH.[19]

3) THE ACCESS FUND   The access fund is intended to support the achievement of NHS Plan targets for patient access to services, in particular reducing waiting times for treatment in accident and emergency departments, and for hospital appointments and admissions. Like strategic capital, the access fund is distributed to SHAs using the same weighted capitation formula used to allocate revenue to PCTs for hospital and community health services (Figure 5.3). £100 million was allocated for this purpose in 2005–6, with the 28 SHAs receiving on average almost £4 million each per annum.[20]

SHAs distribute the access funds to NHS organisations within their areas in such a way as to reward NHS trusts and PCTs which achieve significant improvements in access, for example by paying a certain amount for each percentage improvement in waiting times. For NHS trusts that 'earn' an incentive payment, at least half of it should be spent as decided by the clinical teams responsible for the improved performance. This spending must be on capital items, for example to pay for minor facilities improvements or to replace equipment.

4) PROGRAMME CAPITAL   Programme capital refers to centrally-held budgets for the capital elements in programmes relating to NHS Plan objectives, such as

equipment needed for the improved treatment of cancer. With £2 billion allocated in 2005–6, the single biggest element in programme capital is the information and management technology strategy – part of the National Programme for Information Technology (see Chapter 2, page 23).[21] Programme capital is either distributed directly to NHS trusts and PCTs, or via the SHAs which provide leadership for particular programmes at a regional level.

PROCEEDS FROM LAND SALES AND INTERNALLY GENERATED RESOURCES

As explained earlier, NHS trusts and PCTs 'own' their assets but with an associated 'debt' to the Treasury, known as 'public dividend capital', which they are required to repay if they sell the assets. Repaid public dividend capital, almost all from the sale of land, is used to fund capital projects throughout the NHS; in 2004–5 the sale of assets by NHS trusts and PCTs was expected to raise £102 million, with a further £224 million to come from the sale of assets centrally 'owned' by the Secretary of State for Health.[22] In practice the proceeds of asset sales by NHS trusts and PCTs are retained by the local SHA and used to fund capital development projects within its area. 'High performing' NHS trusts and PCTs are, however, allowed to retain a certain amount of the proceeds of asset sales for re-investment in local services. The amount varies according to the size of their turnover, ranging from £3 million for a 'two-star' organisation (to use the old terminology – see Chapter 6, pages 117–18) with a turnover of less than £30 million, to £10 million for a 'three-star' organisation with a turnover of more than £80 million.[23]

'Internally generated resources' refers to NHS trusts' operating surpluses. Although capital funds can no longer be used to pay for revenue expenditure, the reverse is not true; surplus revenue can be used to fund capital expenditure. It consists principally of surpluses made by NHS trusts from 'selling' their services to PCTs. However, few NHS trusts make sufficient surpluses to fund capital projects significantly; the amount available from this source to fund capital is in practice very limited.

THE PRIVATE FINANCE INITIATIVE

The Private Finance Initiative (PFI) was introduced in 1993 as an alternative to the public funding of capital investment in the hospital and community health services. Although most widely discussed in relation to the building or refurbishment of hospitals by NHS trusts, it is also used by PCTs to fund the development of sites for the provision of community health services, such as rehabilitation and day-hospital facilities. By the late 1990s the PFI had become the major source of capital investment within the hospital and community health services, and formed an integral part of the major capital development programme announced within *The NHS Plan*. Since 1997 PFI schemes worth almost £12.4 billion have been approved, compared with government-funded schemes worth a total of just £280 million. This means that the PFI accounts for 98 per cent (by value) of building schemes in the NHS hospital and community health services.[24]

Under the PFI a private sector consortium of bankers and shareholders raises the finance for capital investment. In return they receive a contract to design and build premises and to operate support services such as maintenance and cleaning. They typically also receive ownership of the assets (land and sometimes buildings), which NHS trusts lease back through contracts, typically of 25 or 30 years' duration. Annual payments under these contracts, which contain both a capital element and an operating element (for the non-clinical or support services supplied by the consortium), are met out of trusts' annual revenue allocations.

Individual NHS hospital trusts or PCTs are responsible for developing proposals for capital development schemes under the PFI, although SHA approval is required. For schemes over £25 million DH approval is also required, and for schemes over £100 million, Treasury approval.[19] Schemes over £25 million also require approval by the Capital Prioritisation Advisory Group (CPAG), a DH body intended to address the need for a strategic approach to the planning of capital investment. In practice its assessments are concerned largely with the financial viability of proposed individual schemes, rather than with the need for such investments,[25] so in some areas SHAs work together to try to provide a more strategic approach.

PRIVATE SECTOR FUNDING OF CAPITAL

The use of independent (private and voluntary) sector healthcare services by the NHS has become an important policy aim of the DH. This involves the use of existing or new, purpose-built capital assets – typically private hospitals or treatment centres – funded by the private sector to reduce the NHS's need for capital. Commercial providers, however, need to be able to make a profit on their investment through the prices charged to the NHS organisations which commission their services. It is unclear whether this will be possible when, as the DH intends, independent sector providers are eventually paid only the same rates as NHS organisations (see page 99).

FOUNDATION TRUSTS (FTS)

As we saw in Chapter 4, foundation status was introduced for NHS hospital trusts in 2004, with the intention that PCTs and even non-NHS bodies will ultimately be eligible to apply for it too. The following discussion, however, relates only to foundation trusts which were previously NHS hospital trusts.

Foundation trusts operate under a different capital framework from that governing NHS trusts. Like NHS trusts they 'own' their assets, with an associated debt to the Treasury (called 'public dividend capital'); but unlike NHS trusts they are able to retain all the proceeds from the sale of assets for re-investment in their own organisations. They do, however, require the approval of the independent regulator, Monitor, to dispose of any so-called 'protected' assets (those deemed by the regulator to be necessary for the provision of NHS goods and services).*

Like NHS trusts foundation trusts can apply to the local SHA for DH funding in the form of 'strategic' capital to support major developments, and can also use the PFI to fund such developments. At the discretion of the Secretary of State for Health they are also eligible for DH funding in the form of public dividend capital, in the form of either loans or grants. Unlike NHS trusts, however, they can also borrow money on the commercial markets. This borrowing is not guaranteed by the Secretary of State for Health, and usually carries a higher interest rate than borrowing from the government. Foundation trusts are able to borrow commercially following a 'prudential borrowing code' determined by the independent regulator (Monitor), who sets an upper limit of borrowing for each foundation trust based on a judgment of its ability to service debt.

The funding of capital for primary care

The total primary care estate is valued at around £2.1 billion. Most primary care premises are privately owned – only 16 per cent are owned by the NHS, whereas 63 per cent are owner-occupied and 21 per cent are leased from private landlords.[26] NHS funds do, however, support the purchase and maintenance of these assets, through the reimbursement of GPs for costs relating to premises and other capital items. It is private finance, however, which now forms the main source of funding for the acquisition of primary care assets, through a variety of forms of ownership, including public–private partnerships.

THE REIMBURSEMENT OF GPs

Although GPs are independent practitioners, under the terms of their contracts they are eligible for re-imbursement from NHS funds for the costs of the primary care facilities they use. This includes financial assistance for items such as business rates, water and sewage, as well as for 'recurring' premises costs. The latter include rent paid on a lease ('leasehold rent') and a prescribed percentage of the interest paid on loans taken out to buy, build or modify premises ('owner-occupier borrowing costs'). If they own a property outright, GPs can claim a payment for its 'notional rent' – i.e. what they would pay if they leased the premises – and they can also receive financial assistance for the cost of leasing medical equipment ('equipment costs'). They can get 'improvement grants' to help with the costs of refurbishing and improving existing premises, both when maintaining their assets and when adding to them, and can claim some of the costs of relocating into modern 'PCT approved' premises, including such items as professional fees and the cost of mortgage redemption or lease surrender. GPs also enjoy a protected minimum selling price for their previous premises, the PCT

---

* According to Monitor, in this context 'assets' refers only to land and buildings. Equipment is exempt.

making up any difference between the protected minimum price and the price actually received.

Separate allocations are made to support the running costs of the existing primary care estate, and to support the costs of new capital development projects, both of which PCTs can supplement from their direct or 'unified' revenue allocations if they deem it necessary.

1) The existing primary care estate

The reimbursement of GPs who claim costs for premises that existed (or whose acquisition had been agreed) prior to the implementation of the new GMS contract in 2004 is paid for out of PCTs' direct unified revenue allocations, which include provision for premises used in primary medical services. In 2005–6, £369 million was allocated for this purpose across England, each PCT receiving the 'historical' level of expenditure within its area, 'uplifted' for the effects of inflation.[27] Expenditure is limited by a requirement that PCTs must approve all premises against a set of 'minimum requirements', such as having properly-equipped consulting rooms, security arrangements for drugs and patient records, and adequate access for disabled patients.[28] Payments are made according to a schedule of 'benchmark' costs.

2) Capital developments in primary care: 'growth monies'

The publicly-funded costs of new capital development projects in primary care are met out of so-called 'growth monies'. These are used to reimburse GPs for capital development projects agreed after the implementation of the new general medical services (GMS) contract in 2004, and to pay for new flexibilities in the use of premises by PCTs, such as PCTs taking over the lease of primary care premises and then sub-letting them to the GPs concerned. Funds for England as a whole are shared between PCTs on the basis of weighted capitation, each PCT receiving a share according to the size of the population it serves, adjusted for a 'market forces' factor intended to reflect the costs of providing premises in different areas. These funds are not allocated directly to PCTs but to a so-called 'lead PCT' in each SHA area. In conjunction with the SHA the lead PCT prioritises the development of premises between and within PCT areas, approving expenditure and then allocating funds accordingly. 'Growth monies' totalling £83 million were allocated in this way for 2005–6.[29]

OTHER CAPITAL ALLOCATIONS FOR PRIMARY CARE CAPITAL DEVELOPMENTS

Capital allocations to fund the development of primary care assets are also made through a number of other public funding streams. For example PCTs are able to bid for a share of the £22 million programme to establish 'one stop shop' primary care centres (where patients can receive a wide range of primary, community, social and pharmaceutical services on one site).

In recognition of the need to update and improve the existing primary care estate £108 million was also allocated between 2004 and 2006 to fund the improvement of existing primary care estate, or so-called 'third party' capital. This was allocated in the form of improvement grants, for GPs wishing to refurbish or raise the standard of their premises, or for refurbishing GP premises owned by PCTs, or buying up land or old GP leases to make new developments possible. This money was distributed alongside the 'growth monies' used to reimburse GPs costs for developments planned after 2004, and was also allocated to a 'lead' PCT to prioritise and allocate in each SHA area.

PRIVATE FINANCING OF THE PRIMARY CARE ESTATE

Development of the primary care estate has long been funded through 'debt finance', whereby GPs have taken out loans to fund new developments and received financial assistance from the NHS to help with the interest and repayments. Such assistance used to be provided by the General Practice Finance Corporation, a statutory non-profit company which borrowed money from the Treasury and lent it to GPs at a commercial rate. The GPFC, however, was sold to the Norwich Union Life Insurance Society in the 1980s, resulting in a switch to the use of private finance. More recently other new sources of finance for capital in primary care have been used. Although few data are held centrally these sources include private healthcare companies and property companies, and even voluntary bodies, all providing premises through a mixture of leasehold, rental and partnership arrangements.[30]

NHS LIFT

The most important new source of primary care capital finance, however, is the government-sponsored Local Improvement Finance Initiative (NHS LIFT), a public-private investment 'vehicle' for financing the development of premises for primary care and the other family health services. The intention is to use it to refurbish or replace 3,000 GP premises, and develop 500 one-stop primary care centres, through the investment of £1 billion of public and private money.[31] Announced in *The NHS Plan* and subsequently legislated for in the 2001 Health and Social Care Act, 42 schemes were in progress across the country by the spring of 2005, with a further nine in the early stages of development. Each scheme consists of facilities providing premises for both GPs and other family health care practitioners, such as dentists and pharmacists, in a single development.

At the local level LIFT operates in the form of public–private partnerships set up as local limited companies known as LIFTCos. Each of these consists of a private sector partner (identified through a bidding process) and a number of minority stakeholders including the PCT, a body known as 'Partnerships for

Health',* one or more local authorities and, where appropriate, GPs and the local SHA. The LIFTCo takes ownership of premises and/or land and is responsible for refurbishing or building premises commissioned by the local health and social care community through a so-called 'local strategic partnering board' consisting of local stakeholders such as the PCT, the local authority, family health service practitioners, voluntary groups, and the SHA. The LIFTCo leases the premises to GPs and other practitioners, and may also provide support services such as cleaning and maintenance as part of the lease. The company also has exclusive rights to provide any new primary care facilities and/or services that may be called for over a 20-year period, so long as the strategic partnering board judges them to be affordable and value for money. If not, the board can look elsewhere. Individual GPs can choose not to participate, remaining owner-occupiers of their own premises, or renting premises from other landlords.

Of the £1 billion intended investment in NHS LIFT, 80 per cent will come from the private sector, with just £200 million of public money made available to start the process;[32] although between 2003 and 2006 a further £3 million of DH funding was earmarked to help PCTs with the project management costs of developing LIFT schemes.[33] The ongoing costs of LIFT, however, i.e. the reimbursement of GPs and other practitioners for the cost of their leases with the LIFTCo, are met out of the allocations PCTs receive to reimburse GPs for the rental costs of premises (described above on pages 92–3).

The flow of funds: from commissioners to providers

Revenue allocated to PCTs flows to NHS trusts and other organisations providing hospital and community health services through the commissioning or 'purchasing' process. The government considers the 'purchaser–provider split' an important lever with which to shift the balance of power within the NHS. Thus the recent structural re-organisation of the NHS has been accompanied by changes in the way in which revenue flows through it. To grasp the significance of these changes a brief description of the transactions involved in commissioning – i.e. contracts and pricing – is first required.

Contracts and pricing

Since the introduction of the NHS internal market in 1991 the providers of hospital and community health services have 'earned' their revenue through contracts with commissioners (now the PCTs). Competition for these contracts is intended to increase efficiency and improve the quality of services. Within the NHS these contracts have traditionally been known as 'service level agreements' or SLAs, not enforceable in law but overseen by the Secretary of State for Health. In the past they usually took the form of block contracts, giving patients access to a

---

* Partnerships for Health is a public–private partnership between the DH and Partnerships UK. It supports the development of LIFT schemes, and provides them with equity.

defined range of services but not specifying a particular volume of work or a price per case. They required little administrative input and were advantageous in relation to services for which it is difficult to predict volumes of work, but they did not offer much incentive to improve efficiency or quality. Less often used were more specific kinds of contract, such as 'cost and volume' contracts, in which commissioners and providers agree a particular volume of work at a particular price; or 'cost per case' contracts based on an agreed cost or price for each case treated. Although these forms of contract can enable commissioners to try to achieve the 'best' (i.e. the cheapest) price, they are only practicable when the categories of care involved can be precisely specified.

The prices charged by providers were supposed to be related to the cost of all the items that entered into the costs of the services in question. The actual prices charged, however, were often simply agreed following negotiations between commissioners and providers in each case. In the late 1990s, however, a National Schedule of Reference Costs began to be published, an annual publication intended to provide a benchmark for commissioners and providers when negotiating contracts. It sets out average costs of services and procedures, gives details of the actual costs in each NHS trust, and ranks the latter against the national average. More recently the schedule has also covered the costs of PCTs that provide services.

The new financial framework: 'payment by results'

A new financial framework known as 'payment by results' was introduced in the 2002 government publication, *Delivering the NHS Plan*. Foundation trusts began implementing it in April 2004; non-foundation NHS trusts will implement it over a three-year period beginning in April 2005. Starting with elective care, by 2008–9 it will cover 90 per cent of all hospital services (including accident and emergency services). Ultimately all payments for services within the NHS will be 'payments by results', including payments for ambulance services, community health services, certain elements of GP services, the work of NHS treatment centres, and services provided to the NHS by all private sector providers.

The payment by results framework is intended to provide incentives to increase the efficiency and quality of services. Through the use of contracts that concentrate on the volume and mix of services, providers will be paid only for services they have actually provided. The national 'tariff', described in more detail below (pages 97–8), is a list of fixed prices for every service, or treatment; the aim is that competition between providers will be based on better quality and efficiency, not on offering lower prices. Providers will compete to attract patients, who will in future be able to choose where to have their treatment, by offering better services.

Contracts

The new financial framework is based on the use of full cost and volume contracts between commissioners and providers. These detail the number of specific treatments that will be carried out, to be paid for at the national tariff rate (described in the next section). Actual levels of activity are to be monitored through an online information system managed by the Secondary Uses Service or SUS.*

For NHS trusts these contracts (known as service level agreements) will remain as NHS contracts, non-enforceable by law but overseen by the Secretary of State. For services commissioned from foundation trusts and the independent sector, legally binding contracts are used. Both kinds of contract should contain explicit arrangements for 'risk sharing'; this is subject to local negotiation, but the DH's intention is that in general the commissioners should 'bear the risk' if they refer more patients than foreseen in the contract, and will be required to pay NHS trusts for the additional services provided. Commissioners will also bear the risk if they fail to refer the agreed number of patients, or prevent the delivery of the planned number of elective services due to having underestimated the number of emergency referrals; in both cases they will receive no reimbursement for the patients contracted for but not treated. Conversely, if providers fail to provide the agreed number of services, despite having patients referred to them, they will bear the risk and have to reimburse the commissioning PCTs or GP practices, at the national tariff rate, for each untreated case.[34] The necessary reimbursements are to take place on a quarterly basis when the state of each contract is reviewed.

As part of the monitoring process the contracts should also specify explicit 'trigger points', levels of activity higher and lower than those agreed within the contract, to alert both commissioners and providers to the need to discuss levels of activity and if necessary take pre-emptive action (5 per cent above or below the planned level of activity is the 'default' difference suggested in the DH's model service level agreement).[35]

Pricing: the national tariff

The new financial framework is intended to ensure that competition between providers is based on the quality of their services (such as length of wait), which depends ultimately on their efficiency (having lower costs and so earning surpluses, and so being able to improve services). Price competition between providers is excluded by the national tariff which sets out a fixed price for every procedure performed by any NHS provider. All PCTs will pay the same prices, irrespective of a provider's location; providers, however, can receive a 'top-up' payment from the DH to cover any extra costs resulting from their geographical location. As an incentive for efficiency, providers who are able to deliver services at a cost below tariff prices will be able to retain the resulting surplus; those unable to cover their

---

* This information system is being developed as part of the national programme for information technology and replaces the 'commissioning data set clearing function' hitherto performed by the NHS clearing service.

costs at the prices set in the national tariff receive no extra funding and so will be forced to cut costs in order to maintain their services (or in the worst case, to avoid being closed down).

Prices within the national tariff are based on those in the NHS schedule of reference costs, the schedule of average prices charged by NHS hospitals and foundation trusts. They include the costs of both clinical and non-clinical items (such as food, maintenance and administration). Since a given provider's 'case-mix' (the mix of health problems patients present, like disease severity, or patients' co-morbidity) can have significant cost implications, prices in the tariff are set for 'health resource groups' (HRGs) rather than for individual diseases or treatments. HRGs are a classification system developed by the former NHS Information Authority, similar to the case-mix adjustment system of 'diagnostic resource groups' or DRGs developed in the USA. For the purpose of the national tariff they classify so-called 'spells' of care (the time from hospital admission to discharge or death) into 'iso-resource groups' – groups of 'spells' for which the cost of diagnosis, treatment and care is similar. For example in 2005–6 a provider would receive £1,489 for a caesarean section without complications, but £2,067 for a caesarean section with complications.[36]

For the hospital services alone there are over 500 HRGs relating to admitted inpatient care; outpatient attendances are classified into 39 HRGs, and accident and emergency attendances into three (high cost, standard and minor injury unit attendance).[35] Elective inpatients and day-case patients are paid for at the same price; this is intended to provide a financial incentive for trusts to provide more services on a cheaper day-case basis where this can be done, involving as it does a much shorter length of stay. Commissioners and providers can also negotiate ways to 'share' certain elements of the tariff price. For example, where the commissioning PCT provides its own post-operative rehabilitation services it can, by agreement with the provider, retain part of the tariff rate to account for this.

Patient choice

Central to the new financial framework is the right of patients, rather than commissioners, to choose their service providers. The intention is that patients' choices will 'drive' the system by linking their choices to financial rewards – paying providers on the basis of work undertaken, so that the flow of funds follows the choices made by patients. This is considered a lever to promote efficiency, making providers compete for patients on the basis of the quality of their services.

The concept of individual patient choice was introduced in 2000 in *The NHS Plan*, which looked forward to patients being able to choose the date and time of hospital appointments and admissions. The 2002 publication, *Delivering the NHS Plan*, subsequently expanded this policy, referring to patients as 'consumers' and declaring that patients' right to choose between hospital providers should become a central feature of the NHS. This was first implemented for patients waiting longer than six months for cardiac surgery, but by December 2005 all patients needing elective care are to be offered the choice of four or five providers.

These may include NHS trusts, foundation trusts, NHS or independent treatment centres, independent sector hospitals and GPs with special interests. By 2008 the policy will be extended further; patients will have the right to choose from 'any healthcare provider which meets the Healthcare Commission's standards, [and] which can provide the care within the price the NHS will pay [the national tariff]'.[37]

In consultation with their GPs patients will choose their provider as well as the date and time of their appointment or admission, on the basis of greatly increased information about the services that are available: the findings of inspections by the Healthcare Commission, performance ratings, and information on waiting times. PCTs will be required to ensure that patients have access to this information and that they get support from GPs, other healthcare professionals and support workers when making their choices.

Contracts with the independent sector

Although the independent sector will ultimately fall within the scope of the new financial framework, in the medium term separate commissioning arrangements are being used. It has been recognised that new units set up and run by the independent sector may face additional 'start-up' costs. This recognition is reflected in higher prices paid to these providers, and contracts of up to five years. At least for the duration of the initial contracts they will be paid outside the NHS financial framework, at prices agreed during the procurement process (the commissioners, however, only pay national tariff prices; the DH uses a central budget to underwrite the procurement process and 'top-up' the difference between the tariff paid by PCTs or commissioning GPs and the higher prices charged by the independent sector). The resulting contracts are made either with the DH (for instance in the case of the services commissioned from the Independent Sector Treatment Centres or ISTCs), or with individual PCTs, and are legally enforceable.

Other sources of funding for providers: cross-charging and joint ventures

In 2002 the government publication *Delivering the NHS Plan* announced the introduction of an additional source of revenue for providers:[38] the 2003 Community Care (Delayed Discharges) Act enabled all NHS trusts, foundation hospitals, and independent sector hospitals providing NHS care to 'cross-charge' local authorities for delayed discharges – i.e. for the daily costs of keeping people in hospital whose discharge is delayed because appropriate non-hospital-based care is not available. The aim is to give local authorities an incentive to provide the necessary alternative care.

This system was introduced in January 2004; hospitals providing acute care (secondary care services, including older people's services) bill local authorities £100 per day (£120 in London) for every patient whose discharge is delayed. To help local authorities respond constructively some NHS funding has been made available to meet these costs while additional facilities are developed; £100 million of NHS money was made available for England in 2004.[39] The intention is that the system of cross-charging will eventually be extended throughout the whole system of care, including services such as mental health services and community care services.

The 2001 Health and Social Care Act also enabled providers to generate funds from commercial sources. NHS trusts and foundation trusts can enter into partnerships or joint ventures with private companies in order to generate income. They can form companies to supply goods or services, or to exploit intellectual property such as marketing technological advances or the findings of research studies, with assets, loans and financial guarantees provided by the NHS.

Financial duties of NHS bodies

As publicly-funded organisations all NHS bodies have a number of financial duties. Under the public sector payment policy introduced in March 1996 they are required to pay their bills promptly: the target set for public sector agencies was to pay 95 per cent of all non-disputed invoices within 30 days of receipt of goods, or of a valid invoice.[40] They are also subject to a number of duties relating to the way in which they balance their accounts. These differ for different NHS bodies, reflecting the historical evolution of the NHS financial regime in response to successive structural reorganisations.

Capital charges

Although more commonly discussed in relation to NHS trusts, and subsequently foundation trusts, the financial duty to pay capital charges applies to SHAs and PCTs too, in relation to their premises and any community sites they may own. The capital charging system was introduced by the 1990 NHS and Community Care Act, and was intended to increase awareness of the costs of capital – the money tied up in assets and not available for use elsewhere – and to provide an incentive for its efficient use.

As we have already noted, while NHS bodies own their capital assets (land, buildings and equipment), they owe a corresponding debt to the Treasury. With respect to this 'public dividend capital' they pay annual interest or 'dividend' to the Treasury; at the time of writing this was a sum equivalent to 3.5 per cent of the value of their net capital assets. They are also required to pay an annual depreciation charge on their assets. Taken together these two payments are known as 'the capital charge'. In effect, this is money that flows from the Treasury to NHS bodies and back to the Treasury, in such a way as to create incentives to use capital efficiently.

Strategic health authorities and PCTs

Under the NHS Act of 1977 SHAs and PCTs have a statutory duty to keep their net overall expenditure within 'cash limits' set for them by the DH.* They also have a statutory duty to keep their total or 'accrued' expenditure within Annual Resource Limits (ARLs) set by the DH. These are set separately for revenue and for capital, and include non-cash items (such as provision for depreciation) as well as cash items, and provision for future liabilities. In 2003–4 all SHAs stayed within their revenue and capital expenditure limits. Forty-one PCTs reported an overspend with respect to revenue, and two on their capital expenditure.[41]

SHAs and PCTs are also expected to achieve annual operational financial balance in resource terms, i.e. to see that their expenditure is matched by their revenue. Following the introduction of resource accounting and budgeting this duty was defined as keeping within annual resource limits 'without the need for unplanned financial support'. This is a 'performance management' measure (see Chapter 6, pages 108–9) rather than a statutory duty. In 2003–4 all SHAs achieved financial balance.[41] So-called 'level four' PCTs, which provide services (such as community health or rehabilitation services) themselves, are also required to recover the full costs of these services from the commissioning organisations. This is equivalent to the break-even duty of NHS trusts, described below.

NHS trusts

NHS trusts were established as semi-autonomous bodies under the 1990 NHS and Community Care Act, and their financial duties differ from those of other NHS organisations. They are expected to break even in each and every year, so that their expenditure is covered by their income. The Act, however, only imposes a *duty* to break even 'taking one year with another'. Although the legislation did not specify how this should be interpreted, the system used by the DH covers a three-year 'rolling' period. When an NHS Trust reports a deficit its financial obligation is met if the deficit is recovered within the following two financial years; i.e. it must break even over a three-year period (or in exceptional cases, a five-year period). In 2003–4 all NHS trusts broke even 'taking one year with another', although 65 reported deficits, totalling £138 million.[41]

Trusts' overall expenditure on capital items is constrained by a duty to keep capital expenditure within a limit known as their Capital Resource Limit (CRL) which is set by the Treasury.† The CRL includes both cash and non-cash items (e.g. depreciation), as well as provision for future liabilities. In 2003–4 all but ten NHS trusts succeeded in staying within their CRLs.[41]

---

* The limit includes some items that are notional sums such as provision for future liabilities, so that an SHA or PCT that gets these sums wrong may find it has exceeded its cash limit even though it has not incurred a cash deficit.
† Under the 1990 Act trusts also have a duty to stay within a so-called External Financing Limit or EFL, which sets a limit on their cash expenditure on capital items.

Foundation trusts

Like other NHS bodies, foundation trusts are required to pay capital charges (see above, page 100). They are not, however, subject to the other financial controls of NHS trusts, such as resource and financing limits. Their only other financial duty, under the 2003 Health and Social Care (Community Health and Standards) Act, is a requirement to perform their functions 'effectively, efficiently, and economically'. But as described in Chapter 6 (pages 112–13), the independent regulator, Monitor, oversees the way in which FTs undertake this duty. Monitor sets each FT a prudential borrowing limit which constrains their overall capital expenditure, and the financial performance of FTs forms a key part of the assessment undertaken regularly by Monitor to ensure that they are complying with the terms of their authorisation.

Audit arrangements

All NHS organisations are required to prepare annual summarised accounts on a resource accounting basis, reporting expenditure against the resource (or revenue) and capital limits set by the DH. These accounts are submitted to Parliament, although different auditing and reporting mechanisms are in place for different NHS organisations.

The annual accounts of SHAs, PCTs, NHS trusts and special health authorities are audited by auditors appointed by the Audit Commission. The auditors are required to give their opinion as to whether each organisation's accounts give a 'true and fair view' of its state of affairs and its income and expenditure. This in turn enables the Auditor and Comptroller General to state whether he has given a 'true and fair opinion' of the summarised accounts described below. Auditors are also required to give a separate 'regularity' opinion on whether the income and expenditure were applied to the purposes intended by Parliament, and whether the organisations' financial transactions conformed to the authority they had for them. As a means of detecting potential problems at an early stage the appointed auditors are also required to refer to the Secretary of State for Health any NHS body which they believe may have made a decision involving unlawful expenditure.

Special health authorities submit their accounts and annual reports directly to Parliament. SHAs, PCTs and NHS trusts, however, submit their accounts to the DH, which summarises them for audit by the Comptroller and Auditor General (the head of the National Audit Office). He or she must certify the summarised accounts, and lay them before both Houses of Parliament along with his or her report.

Different arrangements are in place for foundation trusts (FTs). Their boards of governors are responsible for appointing external auditors, and each FT is responsible for laying its accounts before Parliament. Monitor is also required to prepare an annual report for Parliament, including a summary of the accounts of all NHS FTs.

Banking arrangements

Since the Treasury has to borrow money, any 'spare' NHS funds held in commercial bank accounts, however temporarily, represent a cost to the Treasury. Since April 2002 the Secretary of State for Health has been able to specify where NHS trusts, PCTs and SHAs may hold cash and investments, as well as the maximum amounts that may be deposited. At the time of writing they are required to invest any funds in government accounts, in the Paymaster General's office. NHS trusts are allowed to hold a maximum of £50,000 in other institutions,[42] while for SHAs and PCTs the maximum is £15,000.[43]

The NHS Bank

The formation of an NHS Bank was announced in *Delivering the NHS Plan.*[44] It was established in 'shadow form' in 2003 and replaces the previous system of brokerage between NHS trusts, where those with surplus cash lent it to other trusts. As a 'mutual' organisation of the 28 SHAs, the NHS Bank is currently chaired by the DH's Director of Finance. The intention is, however, that it should in due course be jointly controlled by NHS and external specialists in finance, and operate at arm's length from the NHS.

The aim of the NHS Bank is to maximise the use of resources across NHS organisations and across years. It administers a £152 million special assistance 'mutual fund',[45] which provides grants and loans to NHS organisations facing financial difficulties, particularly for areas of service delivery that address NHS Plan goals. It also undertakes a brokerage role for both capital expenditure and cash, lending unspent allocations to NHS organisations that require short-term additional funding. In addition the Bank provides financial support to NHS trusts which are undertaking major capital developments and which are affected by uncertain revenue streams due to the implementation of payment by results. The Bank provides time-limited financial support during the procurement phase, and for up to five years after the construction, of new capital projects. This is to cover additional revenue costs arising from the development, such as the costs of project preparation, moving existing services to other sites, or operating more sophisticated equipment. The amount of support is based on a national scale related to the size of the development.

6   Efficiency and standards

The NHS is in transition from a public system accountable to Parliament to a market-based system of mixed public and private provision, accountable to an independent regulator. Under both systems efficiency, safety and standards of care have to be assured.

In the past efficiency was assured by direct management and supervision from the centre, through regional and local offices of the DH and through health authorities, and by the public service ethos of NHS employees; while standards were mainly the responsibility of the clinical professions, exercised through the Royal Colleges of medicine and other professional bodies. The NHS was also directly accountable to Parliament for both efficiency and standards.

In a market-based system, by contrast, efficiency is meant to be secured by financial incentives and penalties operating on every organisation within the system.

But competition cannot be allowed to drive uncompetitive hospitals into bankruptcy, or force them to close key services, leaving local populations without. So as with other privatised public services an independent regulator – independent of the government – regulates the working of the market to ensure that as NHS trusts are converted into foundation trusts, and become independent market actors, they are financially viable, and remain so. The office of the NHS market regulator is called Monitor.

The shift to a market-based NHS also means that clinical standards and safety must be secured by external monitoring, audits and sanctions, since there is always a temptation for any organisation facing tough competition to reduce costs by lowering standards. This means that many of the internal mechanisms which assured standards under the former publicly-accountable system are being replaced by external regulation. The most important agency in this respect is the Healthcare Commission, which is responsible for ensuring that all health services are 'fit for purpose' and safe, although the standards it applies in the independent sector are currently different from those applied to NHS facilities.

At present both the old and the new systems for ensuring efficiency and clinical standards are still operating side by side (see Figures 6.1 and 6.2). The Healthcare Commission straddles both. Besides enforcing standards and helping the government to meet its political targets, such as reducing waiting times, it

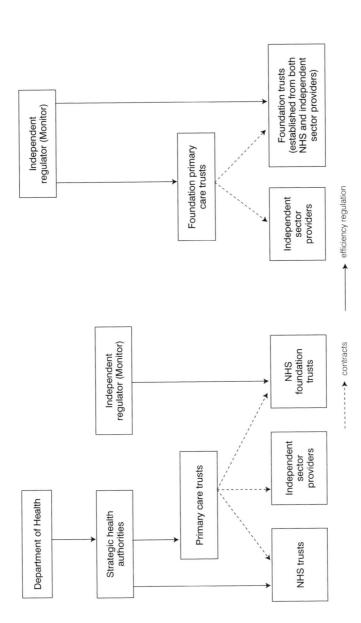

Transition to market (2005)

Full market (circa 2010)* †

Figure 6.1 Securing efficiency in the transition to a market

Notes * All trusts, including primary care trusts, are intended eventually to achieve foundation status and fall under the jurisdiction of Monitor.
† No organisation is currently responsible for regulating independent sector providers, but it has been suggested that non-NHS organisations will be able to apply for foundation status which means they will fall under the jurisdiction of Monitor.

Setting standards

National targets
National standards
National service frameworks
National Institute for Health and Clinical Excellence

Implementing standards

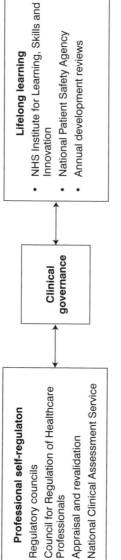

Lifelong learning

- NHS Institute for Learning, Skills and Innovation
- National Patient Safety Agency
- Annual development reviews

Clinical governance

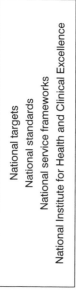

Professional self-regulaton

- Regulatory councils
- Council for Regulation of Healthcare Professionals
- Appraisal and revalidation
- National Clinical Assessment Service

Monitoring standards

Contracts
Strategic health authorities
Healthcare Commission and performance ratings
GP quality and outcomes framework
Patient and public involvement

Figure 6.2 Setting, implementing and monitoring standards in England.

Source: Adapted from A first class service; quality in the new NHS. Department of Health, 1998.

also plays a role in determining the rate at which NHS trusts become ready to enter the market by rating their performance and linking it to financial incentives and penalties. Admission to, and the operation of, the new health care market, in which competition is meant to make all the organisations in it efficient, is the responsibility of Monitor. But the overwhelming majority of NHS trusts are not yet foundation trusts; ensuring their economic efficiency is still the responsibility of the old system of supervision and management, through the Strategic Health Authorities (SHAs). Given that all NHS hospital trusts are intended to become foundation trusts by the end of 2008, the lifespan of the SHAs is presumably limited, but for now they still have a major role to play.

But many other important features of the original system for ensuring efficiency and clinical standards are disappearing. The teams in the DH that used to supervise and manage performance and standards are being disbanded. Some of their functions, including the collection of some information and statistical data, and much workforce and service planning, are disappearing. Others are being absorbed by Monitor and other 'arm's length' bodies concerned with operationalising the new market. Professional self-regulation by the Royal Colleges and other professional bodies is giving way to external monitoring and assessment, and the Royal Colleges' role in setting standards in medical training is giving way to new 'deaneries', over which the government has considerable influence. At the same time new GP and consultants contracts give the government, and increasingly also private healthcare corporations, a large measure of power to determine doctors' methods of working, and the content of their work. And the old structures for public involvement in the NHS are being replaced with consumer models of public engagement, where the focus is on the experiences and concerns of individuals, rather than the general interests of local communities.

The resulting mix of old and new systems and structures of performance management and regulation can seem complex and confusing, and indeed it is; but so long as the essential features of the old and new systems, and the fact that everything is transitional, are kept in mind, the reader should be able to follow the rest of this chapter readily enough.

In practice, of course, 'efficiency' and 'standards' cannot easily be separated. The Healthcare Commission, which is responsible for standards, is concerned with many aspects of the performance of NHS trusts which are 'performance managed' by the SHAs, and the work of the Commission and the SHAs comes together in a system of combined performance 'ratings' which are used to determine the fitness of NHS trusts to achieve foundation status. Likewise Monitor, which is almost solely concerned with financial viability, takes the findings of the Healthcare Commission into account, both in authorising NHS trusts to become foundation trusts, and in regulating their subsequent performance. Nonetheless the broad distinction between issues of efficiency and issues of standards serves as a useful starting-point and the chapter is organised around it, looking first at the mechanisms aimed mainly at ensuring efficiency, and then at those mainly concerned with clinical standards and quality of care.

Contracts

Before looking at the agencies specifically responsible for efficiency and standards, it is necessary first to remember that their work is ultimately grounded on the *contracts* which are integral to the 'purchaser–provider split'. Except for Scotland, all primary and secondary NHS care is delivered on the basis of contracts agreed between purchasers (PCTs or, in some cases, GP practices) and providers – NHS trusts, GPs and independent providers. Within the NHS 'purchasing' actually means 'commissioning', i.e. ordering a given volume of services over a given period. For NHS trusts the commissioning process results in 'service level agreements'. These are not legally enforceable, but the SHAs supervise their fulfilment. For foundation trusts and independent providers, however, legally binding contracts are used.*

The DH intends that the commissioning process should be used by commissioners to hold providers to account for the services they provide. Under the new financial framework described in Chapter 5 commissioning is based on 'cost and volume contracts'. These specify the level of activity to be provided (such as the number of procedures or admissions to hospital), and the cost of each unit of activity (laid down in the national tariff described in Chapter 5, pages 97–8). Activity above or below the specified level requires financial adjustment, and the contracts should also contain explicit agreements regarding the way in which this 'risk' is managed; i.e. who bears the financial consequences of over- or under-activity. If providers fail to provide the contracted number of services, despite being referred the contracted numbers of patients, they 'bear the risk', and are held to account by having to reimburse PCTs for every untreated case. Conversely, if fewer than the contracted numbers of patients are referred, the PCT must compensate the provider.

This system calls for detailed contracts between commissioners and providers, with explicit forecasts regarding the expected or required level of services. It is unclear how it will operate when patient choice is extended in 2008, to give patients undergoing elective procedures the choice of any hospital in England. At the time of writing the way in which the contractual process will be managed, when PCTs will have patients treated at multiple hospitals within England, remains to be clarified.

Strategic health authorities and performance management

SHAs hold PCTs and NHS trusts to account for their financial duties, such as balancing income with expenditure. If they fail to achieve this they are required to produce a financial recovery plan, in conjunction with the SHA. PCTs and NHS trusts are also held to account for their performance in delivering services against

---

*   GP practice contracts with PCTs are also legally binding, although so long as GPs were paid primarily on a fee for service basis, not specified levels of work, this was very seldom significant. As GP practice contracts increasingly specify levels of activity, this may change.

both national targets (discussed below) and local priorities. National targets include issues such as the average time taken from GP referral to a hospital appointment. Local priorities for PCTs might be such aims as improving immunisation rates or reducing inequalities of access; for NHS trusts local targets might be implementing chronic disease management systems or focusing on particular services where problems or potential improvements have been identified. Performance in terms of organisational and workforce development is also assessed, for example against targets for the implementation of GP appraisals, the development of the workforce, or the implementation of the European Working Time Directive and the 'New Deal', which since 2004 have set limits on the working hours and rest periods of doctors in training.

Performance is monitored throughout the year, on the basis of weekly, monthly and quarterly returns made by PCTs and NHS trusts, covering issues ranging from their financial balances to waiting times. There are also regular meetings between the SHA and the 'performance manager' of each PCT or NHS trust, and performance is also formally assessed at least once a year through meetings between the SHA chair and the chief executive of the PCT or NHS trust.

National targets

In 2000 *The NHS Plan* announced the introduction of a 'limited number of ambitious but achievable' targets for the NHS.[1] Targets based on the DH's public service agreement with the Treasury* were subsequently laid out in planning guidance for NHS organisations. In line with the three-yearly allocations of funding to PCTs (see Chapter 5, page 80), targets also relate to three-year periods. Sixty-two national targets were set for the period 2003–4 to 2005–6.[2] In July 2004 a set of new targets for the period 2005–6 to 2007–8 was published, reducing their number to 20.[3] This reduction was intended to create 'headroom' for PCTs to set their own local targets, identifying areas where improvements are most needed at the local level.

Over half of the new national targets to be achieved by 2008 relate to the outcomes of healthcare, rather than to the way in which services are provided, reflecting a greater emphasis on local flexibility in the way services are delivered and targets achieved. They relate to four priority areas: 1) improving the health and well-being of the population, with targets such as reducing mortality rates from heart disease; 2) supporting people with long-term conditions, with targets such as reducing their use of emergency beds; 3) improving access to services, with targets such as ensuring that no-one waits longer than 18 weeks from a GP referral to a hospital appointment; 4) improving the patient or user experience, with targets such as increasing the proportion of older people supported to live in their own homes.

---

* This is the agreement under which the Treasury provides funds to the DH and the NHS, setting out objectives such as improving mortality rates from cancer.

Achievement of national targets is ultimately the responsibility of PCTs, working in co-operation with NHS trusts and other organisations such as the voluntary and independent sector providers from which PCTs commission services. Any contribution by the providers to the achievement of targets should be specified in the contracts PCTs use to commission services. Close co-operation between health and social care organisations has also been recognised as key to achieving these targets, for example through local authorities providing support to older people living in the community.

PCTs, and in some instances NHS trusts, receive dedicated funding to help them achieve national targets, and there are several national initiatives to help them identify and implement 'best practice', and redesign systems of care. Examples include the National Programme for Information Technology (Chapter 2, page 23), which is intended to make it possible to book hospital appointments online and so improve access to hospital appointments for elective care. Achievement of these targets is monitored through a variety of mechanisms, such as surveys by the DH, performance management by the SHAs, and inspections by the Healthcare Commission as part of the performance rating system (see page 116–20).

National standards

Standards differ from targets in being qualitative rather than quantitative. The DH describes them as the level of quality that NHS organisations are expected to meet or aspire to. The 2003 Health and Social Care (Community Health and Standards) Act gave the Secretary of State the power to set national standards for NHS organisations, and in 2004 the DH published a set of 34 standards covering the whole spectrum of NHS care – hospital care, primary and community care, and public health.[4] These standards apply to all bodies commissioning or providing NHS services – PCTs and NHS trusts as well as foundation trusts, and independent sector providers and voluntary bodies with respect to any NHS services they provide. They are also used by the Healthcare Commission to assess the quality of care provided by these organisations, contributing to their subsequent performance rating (see pages 117–20). The DH also intends that these standards will eventually replace these currently used for inspecting the private health services.

The standards published in 2004 are organised in seven 'domains': 1) safety (e.g. following national child protection guidelines); 2) clinical and cost effectiveness (e.g. conforming to NICE guidance – see below pages 113–14); 3) governance (e.g. systems for financial management, or the management of patient records); 4) 'patient focus' (e.g. providing information to patients and their carers); 5) accessible and responsive care (e.g. ensuring that emergency patients are able to access care promptly); 6) the 'care environment' and amenities (e.g. providing well-maintained and clean environments); and 7) public health issues (e.g. the implementation of disease prevention and health promotion programmes).

Each of these domains has a number of both 'core' and 'developmental' standards. The 24 'core' standards are based on existing requirements and describe acceptable levels of service which should be universally achieved. The ten 'developmental' standards are intended to provide scope for continuous improvements in services, making it possible to measure progress year by year. For example the safety domain has a 'core' standard requiring organisations to decontaminate re-usable medical devices properly, and a 'developmental' standard requiring organisations to continuously and systematically review and improve all aspects of their activities that affect patient safety.

Accountability: who is responsible

NHS trusts

Except for trusts with foundation status, the line of responsibility runs from NHS trusts, including PCTs, through the SHAs to the Secretary of State and Parliament.

The boards of directors of NHS trusts are collectively responsible for ensuring that their organisations meet their financial, statutory, and legal responsibilities. NHS boards are led by part-time chairpersons, responsible for ensuring that the organisation discharges its responsibilities as a whole. They have executive members, such as the chief executive and the director of finance, and part-time non-executive members, some of whom are intended to represent the local population. The chief executive is responsible for implementing the board's decisions and for the operation of the organisation. He or she acts as the accountable officer for the board, and is required to produce an annual report and submit audited annual accounts to Parliament via the DH.

Both NHS hospital trusts and PCTs are held to account by their local SHA, by whom they are 'performance managed'. This takes place through an 'annual accountability agreement'. The SHA reviews the performance of each organisation against the agreement, which is based on the targets agreed in the Local Delivery Plan (see Chapter 2, page 19). The SHA determines the performance management framework, setting out which targets should be met and how they should be monitored.

SHAs themselves are held to account by the DH through meetings held at least once a year between the SHA's chief executive and the DH Delivery Group, and through annual appraisals against a 'performance assessment framework'.[5] This is analogous to the performance or star-rating system formerly used to assess other NHS organisations (see pages 117–20). The framework encompasses the SHA's financial balance, its management capacity, and the performance of the NHS organisations in its area – both average performance, and changes in PCTs' and NHS trusts' performance in the Healthcare Commission's ratings table, and their performance against key targets in the Local Delivery Plan. The latter targets focus on service outcomes such as waiting list numbers, numbers of new consultants, and death rates from specific diseases such as cancer.

Using this framework SHAs are classified as 'high performing', 'good performing' or 'challenged'. On the principle of 'earned autonomy', high performing organisations are 'rewarded' by lighter and less frequent monitoring by the DH and by greater financial and operational freedoms, such as freedom to use local Modernisation Agency resources (see Chapter 2, page 24) as they wish. SHAs were originally supposed to have only three-year franchises, on the assumption that they would be temporary bodies, simply helping operationalise the transition to a market. Some of them, at least, now seem likely to have slightly longer lives, and to evolve and change as new structures take root.

Foundation trusts

Foundation trusts (FTs) are ultimately accountable to Parliament, but unlike other NHS bodies they fall outside the jurisdiction of the Secretary of State for Health and the SHAs. They are directly accountable only to Monitor.

Monitor, the independent regulator of NHS foundation trusts, was established in April 2004. In 2003–4 it had 28 staff and operating costs of £2.8 million; both staff and expenditure were expected to more than double by 2006.[6] Its role is to grant 'high-performing' NHS trusts licences to operate as foundation trusts, and then to regulate them to ensure that they stay within the terms of their licences. The terms under which each foundation trust operates are set out by Monitor as 'terms of authorisation'. Monitor's decision to authorise and then to regulate a foundation trust, and its subsequent supervision of its performance, is almost wholly based on economic and financial considerations. Evidence that a trust is meeting healthcare needs, which is one of the elements in applications for foundation status, appears to consist mainly of declarations of support from the PCTs that commission its services, plus the verdicts of the Healthcare Commission (see below, pages 116–20) on the trust's performance in relation to the government's targets and standards.

Monitor sets a 'prudential borrowing limit' which determines how much money each FT may borrow, from the private financial markets as well as from the Treasury. The 'PBL' specifies both its maximum permitted cumulative long-term borrowing and its allowed annual working capital facility for short-term cash flow management.

The ability of foundation trusts to comply with their terms of authorisation is assessed on the basis of 'self-certification' by the foundation trusts themselves, supplemented by reports by third parties such as the Healthcare Commission. Self-certification involves each foundation trust submitting an annual plan to Monitor, which includes its financial management plans; its governance arrangements (such as the membership of the trust, its use of performance management arrangements, and its performance against national standards and targets as assessed by the Healthcare Commission); and its provision of 'mandatory' services as detailed in its terms of authorisation (such as plans for service redesign, or the disposal of so-called regulated assets, as described in Chapter 4, page 64).

Monitor assigns each FT a 'risk rating' for each of these three elements, which measures the risk that the trust will breach its terms of authorisation for that element – in contrast to the Healthcare Commission's performance ratings, which assess the previous year's performance. Risk ratings determine the level of in-year monitoring that Monitor will devote to the foundation trust in question. Those with a 'good' rating are required to submit quarterly, and subsequently six-monthly, reports detailing their performance and how they have complied with their annual plan and their terms of authorisation. In contrast those with the worst risk ratings are subject to in-depth monthly monitoring.

If Monitor deems a foundation trust to be 'significantly' failing to comply with its terms of authorisation it has statutory powers of intervention (although the 2003 Health and Social Care Act did not define what a 'significant' failure is). It may issue warning notices a foundation trust and require a foundation trust to act or cease to act in a certain way. It may also seek an agreement with any creditors for a foundation trust to pay off debts, may replace members of the board of directors or board of governors, and in extreme cases require a foundation trust to cease operation and transfer its assets and liabilities to another NHS body (although this requires the agreement of the Secretary of State and an Order of the High Court). At the time of writing Monitor had used these powers in respect of Bradford Teaching Hospitals Foundation Trust, replacing the chair of the board of directors following a predicted financial deficit of £11.3 million for the year 2004–5.[7]

Clinical standards and safety

Clinical performance has also become the subject of government efforts to establish and enforce national standards, through a combination of four main mechanisms: the National Institute for Clinical Excellence (NICE), also described in Chapter 2, pages 28–9; 'National Service Frameworks' (NSFs) for particular conditions or categories of patient; and 'clinical governance'. Responsibility for ensuring that all NHS organisations follow these regulations lies primarily with the Healthcare Commission. In addition, an extensive overhaul of the healthcare professions is being undertaken.

The National Institute for Health and Clinical Excellence

The role of NICE (as it is still generally called) is to provide health professionals and the public with authoritative and reliable information on evidence-based 'best practice'. Healthcare professionals are expected to take this guidance into consideration when treating individual patients. NHS organisations are also expected to provide funding and other resources for medicines and treatments recommended by NICE, and have three months to do so from the date of publication of NICE's technology appraisals.

Using independent groups or committees of healthcare professionals working in the NHS, and people who are familiar with issues affecting patients and carers, NICE produces and disseminates national guidance on the clinical effectiveness and cost-effectiveness of specific treatments and interventions in three areas: 1) 'technology appraisals', i.e. appraisals of new and existing medicines, treatments, and health promotion activities (such as ways of helping people with chronic conditions to manage their illnesses); 2) clinical guidelines, regarding the treatment and care of patients with specific diseases and conditions; 3) appraisals of interventional procedures for diagnosis and treatment to determine whether they are safe and effective enough for routine use. Each NICE 'guidance' typically takes one to two years to produce.

National service frameworks

National service frameworks (NSFs) are intended to provide 'blue-prints' for the way services are provided by NHS organisations and healthcare professionals, describing the 'quality requirements' for service provision. They are currently being produced for priority areas, i.e. services for major conditions or specific care groups (such as the elderly or children). They are also intended to provide a mechanism through which patients can be clear about what they can expect from the health service.

Addressing the whole system of care, NSFs set explicit standards for service delivery and treatment and define service models in terms of the pattern and level of services required. This includes putting in place programmes to support implementation, and establishing performance measures against which progress within an agreed timescale can be measured. NSFs are developed by the DH, with the assistance of an external reference group for each one. These groups consist of health professionals, health service managers, partner agencies and service users and carers, who meet to review the evidence base and recommend the contents of the NSF in question.

The programme of NSFs was initiated in April 1998, to produce an average of one per year. By Spring 2005 eight NSFs had been published: for mental health (September 1999), coronary heart disease (March 2000), the national cancer plan (September 2000), older people's services (March 2001), diabetes (December 2001 and January 2003), children (April 2003), renal disease (January 2004) and long-term conditions (March 2005).

Clinical governance

Under the 1999 Health Act a duty of quality was imposed upon NHS organisations, requiring them to put in place arrangements to monitor and improve the quality of their services. This was operationalised in the form of 'clinical governance', introduced for all NHS organisations in April 1999. Clinical governance is intended to ensure the continuous improvement of services, as well as the involvement of patients. It has been described as 'a framework through which organisations are accountable for continuously improving the quality of their services and safeguarding high standards of care by creating an environment in which excellence in clinical care will flourish'.[8]

As part of the clinical governance agenda NHS organisations are required to have clear lines of responsibility and accountability for the overall quality of clinical care. Chief executives are accountable for the quality of services on behalf of their boards of directors, and boards designate a senior clinician to be responsible for ensuring that the appropriate systems are in place and are being monitored for effectiveness. Boards can discharge their responsibilities through clinical governance committees, but should receive regular reports on clinical governance arrangements and their effectiveness in the same way that they receive reports on financial matters.

Clinical governance activities are classified into seven areas known as 'pillars' or domains. The first is clinical audit, with departments required to audit their clinical practice on a regular basis. The care provided is assessed against explicit criteria of best practice. Where the need for change is indicated, further monitoring is undertaken to determine the improvement achieved. The second domain is clinical risk management. Organisations should have clear policies aimed at managing clinical risk, systematically assessing it and putting programmes in place to reduce it. Examples include systems for reporting and learning from critical incidents, and clear policies enabling staff to report concerns about their colleagues' professional conduct, and supporting them when they do so. The third area is clinical effectiveness programmes, to ensure the use of evidence-based practice and the implementation of the NSFs and guidance from NICE. The fourth area is education and training and the continuous professional development of staff. Educational courses must be made available to ensure that staff are up-to-date and, when necessary, supervised. The fifth area is staffing and staff management. This area includes issues such as whether systems are in place to ensure the development of staff, whether human resources policies are available for all staff, and whether regular appraisals of staff are undertaken to identify their learning needs and ensure staff competence. The sixth area is the use of information to support quality improvement, for example gathering information on adverse incidents, disseminating the findings of audit projects, and systems to ensure the confidentiality of patient information. The seventh area is patient involvement. Processes should be in place to ensure that patients' views are gathered, and that information from patients, including complaints and surveys of patient experiences, is taken into account when services are planned.

NHS organisations are expected to fund clinical governance arrangements themselves, but a national clinical governance support team, which now forms part of the Modernisation Agency (see Chapter 2, page 24), was established by the DH in August 1999 to provide practical support to clinicians and managers in implementing clinical governance arrangements.

The clinical governance arrangements of individual NHS trusts and PCTs are assessed by the Healthcare Commission. This assessment initially took place as part of a continuous programme of 'clinical governance reviews'; the intention was that each organisation should be reviewed every three to four years. Their performance was examined against the seven 'pillars' of clinical governance described above, along with their strategic capacity (how the organisation led and implemented clinical governance) and patients' experience (to determine what it is like to be a user of the services). Findings were reported to the DH and the relevant SHA, as well as being fed back to the organisations so that they could make improvements.

From 2005–6 onwards, however, clinical governance arrangements are to form part of the governance 'domain' within the DH's national standards, described earlier (pages 110–11). They will be assessed on an annual basis as part of the Healthcare Commission's annual reviews, and will contribute to determining the organisation's performance ratings, discussed in the next section.

Performance 'frameworks' and performance ratings

The Healthcare Commission

As already described in outline in Chapter 2 (pages 30–1), the Healthcare Commission is the product of a merger of the former Commission for Health Improvement, created in 1999, the National Care Standards Commission (which regulated the provision of healthcare provided by the independent sector), the Mental Health Act Commission (which regulated the provision of mental health services and the use of the power of compulsory detention under the Mental Health Act), and the value-for-money work of the Audit Commission.

By 2008 the Healthcare Commission's remit will be extended to cover the inspection of social care providers, both local authority and private and voluntary, through a merger with the Commission for Social Care Inspection (CSCI). (Where appropriate the Healthcare Commission already undertakes joint inspections with the CSCI, for example when inspecting mental health services which involve both a health and a social care element.)

As an executive non-departmental public body the Healthcare Commission is directly accountable to Parliament for improving the quality of healthcare services in England.* It submits an annual report to Parliament on the 'state of healthcare' provision by or for NHS bodies, and also issues various 'national themed reports', for example reports on the implementation of the NSFs and the provision of specific services by NHS trusts. It also examines whether NHS organisations are achieving 'value for money', for example reviewing how efficiently NHS trusts manage their inpatient beds, or facilities such as catering and laundry.

The Commission is also responsible for gathering the views of patients and staff by undertaking national surveys, either on specific services (such as accident and emergency services) provided by individual organisations (including organisations that commission services), or on forms of service, for example surveys of the experiences of inpatients in each NHS trust (patients are asked for their opinions of the local services in primary, community, and secondary care). In addition the Commission reviews patients' complaints which cannot be resolved locally, and investigates 'serious service failures'. Examples of the latter are investigations into charges of bullying or harassment, or into systems of care following a series of adverse events.

---

*   The Healthcare Commission's remit also includes Wales, although with a more limited set of functions.

The Healthcare Commission is probably best known, however, for its role in inspecting healthcare organisations. As discussed above it assesses PCTs, NHS trusts and foundation trusts against the targets and standards set by the DH and awards annual 'performance ratings' (described below) based on the results. When problems are identified the Commission can recommend special measures, such as extra support from, or intervention by, the local SHA, repeat visits, 'franchised' management (see Chapter 4, page 69), or on rare occasions the suspension or closure of a service.

The Healthcare Commission's remit also extends to the independent (private and voluntary) sector, assessing private hospitals, clinics, and hospices, on the services they provide to private patients as well as those they provide for the NHS. They must be registered and licensed by the Commission in order to operate. By 2006–7 independent sector providers will also be awarded performance ratings on the same basis as NHS organisations. The intention is to move towards a system of full cost recovery for this service.*

The performance rating system

The rating and ranking of NHS organisations was first introduced in April 1999 for health authorities.† Known as the national 'performance assessment framework' the rating system assessed performance in six key areas, with the aim of drawing attention to issues that might need further investigation or action. In 2000 *The NHS Plan* announced the government's intention to extend rating and ranking to all NHS organisations, and performance ratings were subsequently introduced as a means of providing a summary of each organisation's overall performance. Making these performance ratings available to the public also allowed the government to fulfil its commitment to provide patients and the general public with more information about their local healthcare services. Performance ratings were introduced for acute hospital trusts in September 2001, and extended to include mental health, ambulance and primary care trusts by 2003.

The Healthcare Commission produces performance ratings on an annual basis. Until 2005 this involved assessing the performance of PCTs and other NHS trusts against key targets set by the DH. Performance against key financial and access‡ targets was combined with their national ranking for performance against three sets of 'focus area' indicators, depending on the organisation§ in question (i.e. a

---

* Independent sector providers pay fees for registration and licensing that are presently set at rates below the cost of the work involved.
† Health authorities were the organisations which at that time commissioned or purchased services for their resident populations, being subsequently replaced by PCTs.
‡ For PCTs, these were targets such as access to a GP within two working days, and for NHS trusts, targets such as the number of patients waiting longer than four hours (total) in Accident and Emergency.
§ For PCTs these were indicators such as mortality rates from cancer, and screening and immunisation rates. For NHS trusts they were indicators such as death rates following particular procedures, and emergency readmission rates.

Table 6.1   Performance rating of NHS organisations in England, 2004–5

Rating	Number of NHS Trusts*	Number of PCTs
Three stars (high performing)	107	58
Two stars	104	157
One star	59	81
Zero stars (poorly performing)	17	7

Source: Healthcare Commission, NHS performance ratings, 2004/2005, London, 2005.

Note

* This refers to trusts providing acute, specialist, mental health and ambulance services; note that some trusts provide both acute and mental health services and so will be awarded two ratings.

trust or foundation trust, or a PCT). In 2004–5, 58 PCTs and 107 NHS trusts were rated as 'high performing' or 'three star', and 7 PCTs and 17 NHS trusts rated as 'poorly performing' and awarded zero stars (Table 6.1).

Since 2005–6, however, the Healthcare Commission has used a new performance rating system. Performance is now assessed in two areas, first according to whether organisations are 'getting the basics right', and second, according to whether they are 'making and sustaining progress'. These are brought together to produce an annual summary performance rating for each organisation, published in September each year, on a scale of 'excellent', 'good', 'fair', and 'weak'. This applies to NHS provider trusts but also to the services of PCTs, whether directly provided by PCT staff or commissioned from other providers.

There are three components to the assessment of whether NHS organisations are 'getting the basics right', which also incorporate the reviews of other bodies:

1   The first component is a public declaration, made by the board of the organisation, of the extent to which an organisation will meet the 'core' standards set out by the DH in 2004, in the seven areas or 'domains' described above (pages 110–11). The declaration must include the findings of the organisation's external (financial) auditors and the views of the 'local health community' on the extent to which the organisation is meeting the standards (the views of the local patient and public involvement forums discussed on pages 129–30 below), the local authority Overview and Scrutiny Committee (page 131 below), and for NHS trusts without foundation status, the views of their SHA. The Healthcare Commission 'validates' these declarations, using other available information such as surveys of staff and patients, complaints data, information from local organisations such as patient forums, hospital, community, and primary care activity data (such as the average length of stay in hospital, the uptake of services such as screening, and prescribing rates by GPs). A random sample of organisations are then visited and inspected, plus those where the validation process has identified potential problems.

2   The second component of whether organisations are 'getting the basics right' is an assessment of performance against national targets to be achieved by 2007 (see pages 109–10 above). The achievement of these targets is assessed using both routine and specially collected data (such as survey findings).

3   The third component of whether organisations are 'getting the basics right' concerns their use of resources, and whether their financial management is efficient and effective. This includes their overall financial position, how well they manage their financial resources, whether value for money is achieved, and whether their financial governance arrangements are effective. For NHS trusts and PCTs the judgment is based on the assessments of the external auditors appointed by the Audit Commission, and for foundation trusts, on the financial submissions they make to the independent regulator, Monitor.

NHS organisations are also assessed against how well they are 'making and sustaining progress' in improving performance. This involves two components. The first is an assessment of how well organisations are meeting the new national targets for the period 2005–6 to 2007–8, published by the DH in July 2004. As described on page 109 above, these are quantified 'levels' of performance (such as the number of patients waiting less than 18 weeks for a hospital appointment) that NHS organisations are required to achieve by a specific date. They are grouped in the four priority areas: improving the health of the population, supporting people with long-term conditions, access to services, and the experience of patients and users. From 2006–7 onwards the performance of organisations against locally-determined targets will also be included: i.e. targets set in conjunction with their partner organisations (for PCTs this includes NHS trusts and local authorities, for NHS trusts and foundation trusts it includes PCTs).

The second component of whether organisations are 'making and sustaining progress' is an assessment of performance against the 'developmental' standards published by the DH in 2004. As described above, these are intended to make possible an assessment of how far improvements in services continue to be made. Performance is assessed through a series of 'improvement reviews', conducted every two or three years, which examine how well an organisation has improved in each area. These reviews focus on particular domains of the developmental standards, for particular conditions, patient groups, or aspects of service delivery (such as services for heart failure, or performance relating to hospital-acquired infections and safety). An important part of the review process is intended to consist of working with the organisations whose performance has the greatest 'potential for improvement'. The Healthcare Commission aims to help them identify problem areas and to share examples of best practice with them, as a result of which the organisation is expected to produce an action plan detailing how it intends to improve its performance.

The first aim of the performance rating is to provide a mechanism enabling organisations to identify areas where service improvement is needed. However the information is also available to healthcare professionals and the public, through the website of the Healthcare Commission. The intention is that this should be used to inform decisions by NHS organisations when commissioning care, and to inform patients wishing to make use of their right to choose their hospital provider for elective care.

But the performance rating system is also used to 'reward' higher-performing NHS trusts and PCTs with financial incentives. This is known as the system of 'earned autonomy'. Under this system high-performing NHS hospital trusts (previously 'three-star', now 'very good') can apply to Monitor to gain the extra freedoms that come with foundation status. In time PCTs and care trusts will also be able to apply (as well as organisations from the independent sector, see Chapter 4, page 64).

High-performing NHS trusts and PCTs can also gain greater operational and financial freedoms short of full foundation status. These include easier access to capital, freedom to undertake capital projects of greater value without approval from the SHA or the DH, and the right to retain more of the proceeds from any sales of their assets. They can also become subject to less frequent monitoring and inspections, may provide fewer 'returns' detailing their activities and financial situation, and meet less frequently with the SHA as part of their performance management.

They can also get additional freedom to establish 'spin-off' companies or joint ventures with the independent sector to generate income, for example through the exploitation of intellectual property rights. High-performing organisations which already have one such venture approved by the DH are able to undertake additional ventures without requiring DH approval. Achieving the highest performance rating also grants NHS trusts and PCTs automatic entry to the DH's 'register of expertise', which allows them to bid for 'franchises' to manage other NHS organisations, taking over the management of persistently failing PCTs or NHS trusts.*

Conversely poorly-performing organisations become subject to closer monitoring by their SHA. They are also subject to targeted interventions to help them improve services. This can include external support for specific functions or services, for which the poorest-performing trusts are required to produce 'action plans' within three months of their performance rating. They have up to a year to demonstrate improvement; those deemed by ministers to be persistently failing then become eligible to be 'franchised', their senior management being replaced by that of a higher-performing PCT, NHS trust, foundation trust, or independent sector provider, from the DH's 'register of expertise'. In 2001 six NHS trusts had their senior management teams replaced by experienced NHS managers, and in 2003 one had its senior management team replaced by a private sector provider (Secta Group Ltd).[9]

---

* The legal power enabling the DH to require individual NHS organisations to change their senior management was contained in the 2001 Health and Social Care Act.

General practice: the 'quality and outcomes' framework

For general practice the assessment of healthcare is undertaken within the 'quality and outcomes framework' introduced as part of the new General Medical Services contract in April 2004. As described in Chapter 5 (pages 86–7), individual GP practices are awarded 'quality points' for both aspiring to and achieving certain levels of performance.

Performance in four areas is examined by PCTs, in discussion with each practice:

1 the provision of specific services for particular conditions such as coronary heart disease;
2 the provision of 'additional services' such as cervical screening;
3 organisational matters such as the keeping of up-to-date patient summaries; and
4 measures of the 'patient experience', such as the average length of consultations.

This system differs in two key respects from the way in which healthcare provision is assessed for PCTs and NHS trusts. First, it is a voluntary system: GP practices can choose which areas of healthcare provision they wish to be assessed on. Second, it is linked to financial remuneration: practices receive payments according to their performance. £1 billion was allocated nationally for this purpose in 2005–6.[10]

Professional regulation

Self-regulation by the medical professions has been a long-standing tradition in the NHS, involving a system of regulatory councils which provide certification and licensing of practitioners within the UK and hold registers of all those licensed to practice (in both the NHS and the independent sector). As statutory bodies they are responsible for defining standards of education, clinical performance and professional conduct. They also investigate and discipline practitioners about whom there are concerns regarding their clinical practice, professional conduct, or fitness to practice, and have power to terminate a practitioner's licence to practise and remove him or her from the register. They have traditionally been large bodies dominated by professional members, operating their own regulatory and disciplinary procedures. They have functioned more or less autonomously, with various accountability arrangements, some being accountable to the Privy Council (in effect to ministers), and some to the Secretary of State for Health; some have lacked any direct accountability.

The role of the regulatory councils is supported by their corresponding Royal Colleges, established under Royal Charter to encourage education and knowledge in their respective fields, covering all the principal hospital-based clinical specialities such as physicians, surgery, paediatrics, nursing and midwifery, as well as general practice. They have varying roles in setting educational standards and approving educational posts. Like the regulatory bodies their accountability arrangements are also varied, again including accountability to the Privy Council, the Secretary of State for Health, or no direct accountability.

A number of high profile scandals relating to the performance of doctors, such as that which led to a public inquiry into paediatric heart surgery at Bristol Infirmary, which reported in 2001, led to reform of the regulatory councils, the establishment of a National Clinical Assessment Service, and the introduction of a system of appraisal and revalidation for doctors.

Reform of the regulatory councils

In 2000 *The NHS Plan* outlined the government's intention to strengthen the regulatory councils through changes in their constitutions, structures, and internal governance arrangements, to make their procedures more transparent and develop meaningful accountability mechanisms to both the public and the health service. The councils have become smaller bodies, with a greater involvement of the public. For example the General Medical Council (GMC) for doctors has been reduced from 105 members to 35, of whom 19 are doctors (elected by all those licensed to practice), two are academics appointed by universities and the Royal Colleges, and 14 are members of the public appointed by the Privy Council.[11] The latter are known as lay members, and now play a significant role on the disciplinary panels that determine the fitness to practice of individual practitioners.

A new body to oversee the work of the regulatory councils was also established in April 2003, under legislation provided in the 2002 NHS Reform and Healthcare Professions Act. This body, the Council for Healthcare Regulatory Excellence, has 19 members, one appointed by each of the nine regulatory councils and ten lay members. It is responsible for overseeing the work of the regulatory councils, requiring them to conform to the principles of good regulation and providing a mechanism for greater co-ordination, integration and sharing of good practice. It monitors the performance of the councils and can enforce changes in their rules. It also has the right to refer to the High Court any decision by a professional regulatory council that it judges 'unduly lenient' and harmful to the protection of the public. Although the Council is funded by the DH it operates independently and is accountable to Parliament, to which it reports annually. The Council meets in five public and five closed sessions each year in order to review cases. Between September 2003 and the end of October 2004 the Council was notified of 526 cases, 13 of which were referred to the High Court.[12]

The National Clinical Assessment Service (now part of the National Patient Safety Agency)

New mechanisms to address the performance of individual doctors were also outlined in the DH's 1999 publication *Supporting Doctors, Protecting Patients*. These included the establishment in April 2001 of a National Clinical Assessment

Service (NCAS) as a special health authority. As described in Chapter 2 (page 27), its functions were absorbed by the National Patient Safety Agency (NPSA) discussed below (page 126) in April 2005.

The NPSA's remit covers doctors in England and Wales, and since April 2005 also all NHS dentists in England, Wales and Northern Ireland. As an advisory body it provides support to NHS trusts and PCTs in dealing with concerns over the clinical performance of individuals. As the independent sector is increasingly used to provide NHS care, the Agency's remit will presumably be extended to include private and voluntary organisations too. Senior members of these organisations are able to refer their concerns to the NPSA, which uses senior and specially trained doctors, dentists and managers to provide a performance assessment of the clinical practice of the individual practitioner in question. It then provides practical recommendations to the referring body to help resolve any problems identified, such as targeted education, re-training, and/or referral to the GMC. In exceptional circumstances, where the public is felt to be at risk, the NPSA may refer professionals directly to the GMC or the General Dental Council.

By 2005 over 1,200 requests for support and advice had been received.[13] A review of its work during its first 21 months showed that it received 446 referrals regarding doctors, predominantly from the older age groups, 80 per cent of them men, the highest number being in the surgical specialties.[14]

Appraisal and revalidation

The government's 1999 publication *Supporting doctors, protecting patients* also outlined the introduction of a system of annual appraisal for doctors employed in the NHS. It was introduced for hospital consultants in April 2001, and extended to GPs in April 2002, and finally to non-consultant career grades doctors (see Chapter 8, page 150) in September 2003.

Chief executives of NHS trusts, and for GPs, the chief executives of PCTs, are responsible for ensuring that annual appraisals are undertaken. While appraisal does not apply to independent sector providers, NHS doctors undertaking private practice should include information relating to their private practice within their NHS appraisal so that 'whole practice appraisal' is achieved. The DH is also considering how to extend the appraisal process to locum doctors.

The appraisal process is intended to review doctors' performance in the previous year, as well as identifying professional objectives for the coming year within a personal development plan. Annual appraisals are carried out by a fellow professional who is acquainted with the areas of specialist practice of the doctor being appraised. Appraisal is based on the standards of good medical practice produced by the GMC – good clinical care, maintaining good medical practice, teaching and training, relationships with patients, working with colleagues, probity, and health. Those being appraised are required to complete a 'folder' of documentation, providing data on their clinical performance, activities related to training, education, research and audit, how they apply any relevant clinical guidelines, their relationships with patients and colleagues, any concerns or serious clinical complaints regarding their practice, and their personal and organisational effectiveness.

It was initially intended that the annual appraisal process would be supplemented by a five-yearly revalidation process, with doctors wishing to maintain their licences and continue in practice required to present evidence to the GMC every five years showing that they are competent and have kept up-to-date. Validation was due to be implemented in the Spring of 2005, based on the information provided by doctors in their preceding five annual appraisals. However, the fifth and final report of the inquiry into the activities of the GP serial killer Dr Harold Shipman* recommended a much more rigorous revalidation process, including measures such as a knowledge test, video-tapes of consultations with patients, and ratings such as 'pass' or 'fail'. In the spring of 2006 both the process used for revalidation and its date of introduction were still under review.

Ongoing reform

Safeguarding patients also made a number of recommendations relating to other areas of professional regulation. These included the disciplinary procedures available to PCTs for GPs whose conduct is not so problematic that it requires referral to the GMC, but which is nonetheless felt to be unsatisfactory; and the way in which referrals are made to and managed by the GMC (including a recommendation that fitness to practise judgments should be made by a body other than the GMC altogether). It is likely that a number of further changes to professional regulation will be introduced over the coming years.

Lifelong learning

The government's quality agenda also includes the aim of lifelong learning by both individuals and organisations. Two organisations have been established to support this, the NHS Institute for Learning Skills and Innovation, and the National Patient Safety Agency. In addition all NHS staff, other than NHS trust board members, doctors and dentists, are covered by a system of annual development reviews.

The NHS Institute for Learning Skills and Innovation (NHS ILSI)

The Institute was established in July 2005 (see Chapter 2, pages 24–5). It is responsible for developing material to help individual practitioners, teams, and organisations in their everyday work, as well as taking forward the work of the two earlier organisations it absorbed, the Modernisation Agency and the NHS University.

The Modernisation Agency was established in April 2001. Focused on service delivery, its two main roles were to help in modernising services to ensure that

---

* *The Shipman Inquiry, fifth report: Safeguarding Patients: Lessons from the Past – Proposals for the Future*, London: The Stationery Office, 2004.

they met the needs and convenience of patients, and to develop current and future NHS leaders and managers. It also played a central role in the performance improvement programme for NHS organisations, which was intended to enable every NHS hospital trust to achieve foundation status by 2008, and to help every PCT develop its capacity and raise its performance. The agency used staff drawn on secondment from within the NHS, functioning through regional and local teams working with local organisations. It was responsible for a wide range of initiatives.

An NHS leadership centre promoted leadership development, teaching corporate and management skills to clinicians, managers and non-executive lay members of NHS boards, to enable them both to meet their own responsibilities and to take on additional roles such as involvement in PCT professional executive committees, or to progress up the career ladder. A 'new ways of working' team focused on workforce development, looking at ways of redesigning roles and responsibilities, and a clinical governance support team helped trusts and PCTs address poor clinical governance reviews. An innovation and knowledge group supported national and local efforts to modernise services, and a 'technology in health' group supported SHAs in implementing the national programme for information technology (see Chapter 2, page 23). The National Institute for Mental Health in England (NIMHE), which came under the Agency, worked to help local organisations improve and co-ordinate services for people with mental health problems.

The National Primary Care Development Group, an affiliate of the Modernisation Agency, was established to support PCTs and GP practices in improving services, for example through leadership programmes and programmes aimed at improving services for specific conditions such as coronary heart disease and falls by older people. A national primary care and care trust development team (NatPaCT) was also established to work with PCTs and care trusts, to provide support and the opportunity to share and learn from examples of good practice. A service improvement team was established to help improve access to services, for example working with NHS trusts to increase the use of day surgery and implement electronic booking for hospital appointments. A partnership development group focused on integrating the agency with its partner organisations.

With the formation of the new NHS Institute for Learning Skills and Innovation the Modernisation Agency was dissolved. Much of its work was devolved to local NHS organisations, leaving a smaller national modernisation resource within the new Institute. Its role is now to undertake 'diagnostic analyses' of specific service problems, and help design new service improvement programmes.[15]

The NHS University (NHSU), also absorbed by the NHS ILSI, began piloting programmes and services in November 2003, aimed at all staff working in health and social care in England. It offered face-to-face learning as well as 'distance learning' on an internet-based 'virtual campus'. Subjects range from the generic, such as communications skills, or the use of personal development toolkits, to subject-specific matters such as the pre-operative assessment of surgical patients. The NHSU also secures formal learning opportunities for staff in universities, colleges, and has academic partnerships with a number of universities, including the Open University.

The National Patient Safety Agency (NPSA)

In 2000 the DH published *An Organisation with a Memory,* recognising the human and financial costs of adverse events within health care. This led to the establishment in July 2001 of the National Patient Safety Agency (NPSA) as a special health authority, which became operative across the NHS in England and Wales in 2003, absorbing the functions of the earlier National Clinical Assessment Service (described on pages 122–3 above).

Its purpose is to improve patient safety by reducing the risk of harm from medical errors through the promotion of a culture of learning from adverse events. The NPSA operates a national reporting system for adverse healthcare events. This takes place currently through the local reporting systems of NHS organisations, but staff will eventually be able to report adverse events directly through an internet-based system. The NPSA also encourages staff to report incidents without fear of reprimand or reprisals, and also encourages patients and carers to report incidents causing unnecessary suffering or harm. Safety data are also collected from other sources, including patient groups, clinical experts and coroners.

Data are held anonymously (since the NPSA is not responsible for investigating individual incidents), and disseminated across the country via a national reporting and learning system (NRLS) that is currently being implemented across the NHS, using 'root cause analysis', a retrospective review of incidents used to determine what happened, how, and why. Findings are used to identify risks and to produce solutions and measures intended to reduce the risk of further incidents. These findings and solutions are fed back to the organisation concerned, as well as being disseminated across the NHS in the form of safety information, advice and protocols. The NPSA also offers resources such as learning tools for NHS staff to help raise awareness of patient safety issues.

The work of the NPSA is supported by 17 clinical specialty advisers, appointed directly by the NPSA or by one of the Royal Colleges.[16] Their role is to raise the profile of patient safety within the Royal Colleges, and to provide a clinician's viewpoint on how best to ensure the flow of information about adverse incidents and solutions, between their specialty and the NPSA.

Annual development reviews

In October 2004 a system of pay re-structuring was introduced for non-medical NHS staff known as 'Agenda for Change', under which all NHS staff except NHS trust board members, doctors and dentists undergo annual development reviews. In discussion with their reviewer (usually their line manager), individual staff members review their professional activities against the requirements of their posts, with an emphasis on how far they have demonstrated the application of knowledge and skills in practice. They then identify how best to maintain their current level of knowledge and skills, and how to address any gaps which call for further learning. These aims are agreed in a written personal development plan or PDP for the following year.

The requirements of each post are identified, using the NHS 'knowledge and skills framework' or KSF, a classification system which details the skills and knowledge required for any given post, so that every post in an NHS organisation has a KSF outline. The outline has six 'core' dimensions applicable to all positions within the NHS, such as communication skills, and 24 dimensions relating to specific work areas, such as management skills, or other particular kinds of knowledge required for the job.

Patient and public involvement in health care

In *The NHS Plan* the government stated its belief that patients and citizens should have more influence within the NHS,[17] and followed this up with a series of reforms intended to increase the patient and public involvement in health care, and to increase the accountability of NHS organisations to the public.

The 2001 Health and Social Care Act placed a duty on SHAs, PCTs and NHS trusts to make arrangements to involve and consult patients and the public in service planning, the operation of services, and the development of proposals for change, and the 2002 NHS Reform and Healthcare Professions Act spelled out a new system for doing so. While Community Health Councils,* previously known as the independent 'watchdogs' of the NHS, have been abolished, greater lay representation on the boards of directors of NHS organisations is now required, and a system intended to create a partnership between the NHS, patients and the public has been developed under the general oversight of an interim national body known as the Commission for Patient and Public Involvement in Health (described below, pages 128–9). There are also local arrangements for NHS bodies, including oatient and public involvement forums, Patient Advice and Liaison Services, Independent Complaints Advocacy Services, and local authority Overview and Scrutiny Committees. Much more information, both for and from patients, is also part of the process.

Lay representation on NHS boards

Strategic health authorities, PCTs and NHS trusts

The boards of SHAs, PCTs, care trusts and NHS hospital trusts are all required to have lay chairpersons and majorities of lay members, all of whom should live

---

* Community Health Councils were statutory independent bodies drawn from the local community, which NHS bodies were required to consult over any proposed major changes to local services.

locally and use NHS services.* The board of a PCT or an NHS trust must also have a member drawn from its patient and public involvement forum (discussed below, pages 129–30).

Lay members are expected to use their local knowledge and skills to help boards develop strategy, but also to hold boards to account and ensure that the interests of patients and the public remain paramount in policy-making. Since April 2001 they have been appointed by the NHS Appointments Commission, rather than the Secretary of State. As described in Chapter 2 (pages 31–2), the Appointments Commission is responsible for the open and transparent appointment of lay or non-executive directors, following criteria laid down by the Secretary of State.

Foundation trusts

Like other NHS organisations, foundation trusts must have non-executive or lay members on their boards of directors, one of whom should also be the chair, although there need not be a lay majority. Non-executive directors must be drawn from the population served by the foundation trust, or be former or current patients. In foundation trusts, however, they are appointed by the internal mechanism discussed below, not by the NHS Appointments Commission.

Foundation trusts have a system of 'members' and 'governors' that is intended to increase the influence of patients and the public in their management, as well as accountability to patients and the public. As described in more detail in Chapter 4 (pages 65–6), members are drawn from among local residents (the public constituency), past and current patients (the patient constituency), and the staff of the trust (the staff constituency). They should be consulted on matters relating to the provision of services, may stand for election to the board of governors, and elect a majority of the members of the board of governors. The board of governors also contains representatives of other bodies, such as the local authority and the local PCT. The board of governors represents the views of members within the decision-making process by appointing the chair and other non-executive directors to the board of directors, working with the directors to ensure that the foundation trust meets the terms of its licence to operate, and feeding back information about the trust's performance and service development through meetings with the members of whichever 'constituency' they represent.

The Commission for Patient and Public Involvement in Health

The Commission for Patient and Public Involvement in Health (CPPIH) was established in January 2003 under legislation provided in the 2002 NHS Reform and Health Care Professions Act. It became an interim body following the DH

* Strategic health authorities, PCTs and traditionally NHS trusts serve their local geographically defined populations. But the new right of patients to choose their provider of elective secondary care services means that the geographic areas from which the patients of NHS trusts come are likely to become less clear.

review of arm's length bodies (*Reconfiguring the Department of Health's Arm's Length Bodies*), and was due to be abolished in August 2006. It is discussed briefly here since current policy and other documents still refer to it and its functions.

The CPPIH was an 'executive non-departmental public body' – a national body funded by the DH to perform specific functions on behalf of the NHS. In 2003–4 it had some 150 staff and annual operating costs of £24 million.[18] Directly accountable to Parliament, its ten commissioners were appointed by the NHS Appointments Commission. Its role is to support and facilitate effective patient and public involvement throughout the healthcare system.

At national level this involves advising the Secretary of State for Health on mechanisms for patient and public involvement, and carrying out national reviews of services from the patient's perspective. It also has the power to make reports to other bodies such as the Healthcare Commission or the National Patient Safety Agency on patient and public involvement issues and issues that in its opinion give rise to concern about the safety or welfare of patients. Most of its work, however, is at local level, working through a network of contracted 'forum support organisations' to establish, fund, appoint staff to, and oversee the work of patient and public involvement forums.

Patient and public involvement (PPI) forums

The 2001 Health and Social Care Act placed a duty on the Secretary of State to see that a patient and public involvement forum is established in PCTs and NHS trusts. In 2004 there was one for every PCT, NHS trust, and foundation trust, making a total of 572 forums in England.[19] However their numbers are to be reduced through the merging of all the forums within each PCT area into a single forum, whose role will be to monitor the functions of the PCT as well as each of the NHS trusts in its area. This is time-tabled for some time after the summer of 2006.

Patient and Public Involvement Forums (PPI forums) are independent statutory bodies; although currently linked to PCTs, NHS trusts and foundation trusts, they are established under separate legislation and have specific duties and functions. They are required to have ideally ten, but at least seven, members, most of whom must be people who are using or have used the relevant organisation's services, or who live in the area served by the PCT.[20] Other members are drawn from the public and from members of voluntary agencies representing patients or carers. Members are volunteers, appointed by the NHS Appointment Commission. They are expected to represent the views of the public as well as patients, acting as a 'conduit' for the views of the community. They gather the views of patients and carers through surveys and public meetings, and make reports and recommendations about services to their associated trust. Trusts must respond, detailing what action will be taken (or if no action is to be taken, explaining why). PCT forums also have a role in encouraging the involvement of the public in consultations by the PCT, the local SHA, or any NHS trusts or foundation trusts from which it commissions services.

Forums have the power to request relevant information from NHS bodies, and to enter and inspect any premises owned by the trust – in the case of PCT forums this power of entry extends to organisations providing services to the PCT, including NHS trusts and foundation trusts, primary care providers such as GPs and dentists, local authority social services, and independent sector (private and voluntary) services. They can refer any matters relevant to the forum's function to local authority Overview and Scrutiny Committees (see page 131 below), or other bodies such as the Healthcare Commission. A forum member also acts as a non-executive member of the board of directors, representing the views of patients and the public.

Patient advice and liaison services

The 2000 NHS Plan announced the introduction of NHS-wide patient advocacy and liaison services.[21] Following consultation it was decided to separate advice and liaison services from advocacy services (supporting patients and their families who express concerns with services). Patient Advice and Liaison Services (PALS) were introduced for NHS trusts, foundation trusts and PCTs in April 2001, although what is officially acknowledged to have been 'patchy' development has resulted in the establishment of a National PALS Development Group to support their development in SHA areas.

The role of PALS is to provide confidential advice and support to individual patients, carers and their families. This includes giving them information on local health services and putting them in touch with relevant voluntary organisations and support groups. They also inform patients and their families of complaints procedures, putting them in touch with independent complaints advocacy services (described below) if they wish to complain. But one of the roles of PALS is to provide information and advice in the hope of resolving concerns quickly, liaising with clinical staff and managers to prevent concerns escalating into problems or complaints. PALS also monitor problems and submit anonymised reports to NHS trusts and foundation trusts, PCTs, and PPI forums, acting as a form of 'early warning' system.

PALS should be situated in main hospital reception areas and primary care settings, and also be accessible via free-phone numbers, advertised locally. They operate as part of local networks, operating across the boundaries of organisations such as PCTs and NHS trusts. PALS are provided by and responsible to the relevant trust, and their work is monitored for quality and effectiveness by the trust's PPI Forum.

Independent complaints advocacy services

The 2001 Health and Social Care Act required the Secretary of State for Health to provide independent complaints advocacy services (ICAS) for the NHS. These were established in September 2003 on a regional basis under contracts with the

DH.* In the first year of operation the services were provided through 49 offices by 103 advocates or case workers and 55 'client support workers', at a cost of £6.8 million.[22]

The ICAS provides services to individual patients and their carers. Its role is to ensure that they have access to independent assistance and support when making a complaint about NHS services (the NHS complaints procedure is discussed below on pages 132– 4). This includes helping clients to deal with problems they have had with services and identifying the options for taking forward their complaints. Should a client decide to proceed with a complaint the ICAS also supports him or her with any needed assistance, such as help with writing letters or attendance at meetings with a view to making the complaint 'effective'. In its first year of operation the service supported 10,422 complainants.[22] Anonymised information about complaints is also made available to PPI forums to alert them to potential problem areas, and the numbers and kinds of complaints in each region are also reported to the DH.

Overview and scrutiny committees

The 2001 Health and Social Care Act extended the powers of local authorities with respect to NHS services. Since January 2003 local authority overview and scrutiny committees, consisting of elected councillors who oversee the provision of local social services, have also had the power to review and scrutinise local NHS services. This is intended to enhance local authorities' role in improving health and reducing health inequalities, as well as increasing the accountability of NHS services to the public.

These committees are empowered to scrutinise the ongoing planning, operation, and performance of local health services, focussing on the provision of specific services as well as wider issues such as trusts' 'financial recovery' plans (typically involving budget cuts) and their effects on services. They also scrutinise planned major changes in services, which strategic health authorities, PCTs, NHS trusts and foundation trusts must refer to them. They receive reports on patients' views of services from PPI forums, and can call on NHS managers to provide them with information about services and decisions. They report their findings locally, to SHAs, PCTs, and NHS trusts or foundation trusts, as well as other NHS organisations such as PPI forums and the public. They also have the power to refer contested service changes to the Secretary of State. Unlike Patient and Public Involvement Forums, however, Overview and Scrutiny Committees are not funded or otherwise supported by the Commission for Patient and Public Involvement, so it is not clear how far their legal powers will be matched by the practical capacity to exercise them.

---

* The organisations providing services are the Citizen's Advice Bureau, the Carers Federation, POhWER, and the South East Advocacy Projects.

Patient information

Local accountability depends on local communities being well informed about standards and about the services in their area. Good information is also recognised as necessary to enabling patients to make informed choices about where to go for primary and elective secondary care services.

Since 2002 PCTs have been responsible for publishing annual 'patient prospectuses', providing detailed information on their local PCT and on each of the main local health care providers. Prospectuses should include information on the pattern and availability of local services, such as the availability of women GPs, as well as on their quality and performance, including findings from reviews by the Healthcare Commission. They should also contain feedback from patients using local services, including a summary of the patients surveys undertaken annually at the local NHS trust or foundation trust, and of patients' complaints about services.

Patient surveys

Annual nationwide surveys of NHS patients were introduced in the 1997 white paper, *The New NHS: Modern, Dependable.* They were conducted every year between 1998 and 2002, aiming to record patients' experiences of NHS care with a different theme each year, such as services for coronary heart disease. In 2002 they were replaced by a system whereby individual NHS organisations ask patients and carers for their views on the services they have received. These should be included in each organisation's annual prospectus, fed back to PPI forums, and used to identify areas for service improvement. They also contribute to the organisation's annual performance rating. The process is now overseen by the Healthcare Commission: it provides a standard survey procedure as well as collating the findings of the local surveys to produce national themed reports.

Complaints and clinical negligence

Although the NHS's complaints and clinical negligence systems are not strictly part of the regulatory framework, they nonetheless act as constraints on unacceptable performance and are discussed here for the sake of completeness.

Complaints

Complaints regarding NHS services have risen over recent years. In 2003–4 there were over 43,000 written complaints regarding family health services (GPs, and NHS dentists, pharmacists and opticians), and over 90,000 written complaints regarding hospital and community health services.[23] Following a review of the NHS complaints procedure in 1999–2000 the DH set out proposals for reform in the 2003 document *NHS Complaints Reform – Making Things Right.* The Health and Social Care Act 2003 gave the Secretary of State the power to make provision for the handling of complaints, and implementation of the proposals began in 2004. Further reforms may well occur, particularly for primary care practitioners, following the findings of the inquiries into the GP serial killer Harold Shipman.

The NHS complaints system applies to all services provided by NHS organisations or primary care practitioners (GPs, NHS dentists, and pharmacists and optometrists providing NHS services). It also applies to foundation trusts and independent sector providers of NHS services. It does not provide financial compensation to complainants, and cannot be used by people taking or intending to take legal action with respect to a complaint, being based on the principle of 'local resolution'. Complaints should be made directly to the organisation or primary care practitioner providing the service complained of. Foundation trusts and independent sector providers providing NHS services should have their own internal complaints procedures. However NHS bodies such as strategic health authorities, NHS trusts and PCTs, as well as primary care practitioners, are required to use the following procedures.

They must have in place systems to handle and consider complaints and must make patients and their carers well aware of them. NHS trusts should also have a senior member responsible for ensuring compliance with complaints procedures, and a designated complaints manager to handle and investigate complaints. The number and type of complaints should be reviewed on a quarterly basis by the trust's board, and be included in an annual report on the handling of complaints. For primary care practitioners each practice should nominate a member of staff to handle and consider complaints. They should also be able to provide information to their PCT on the number and types of complaints at the PCT's request.

Patients or their representatives can make a complaint, either written or oral, within six months of an incident coming to light. They should receive a written response within ten working days of making a complaint to a primary care practitioner, and within 20 days of making a complaint to an NHS body.[24] The response should summarise the complaint, describe what investigations have been undertaken and their conclusions, and detail the right of the complainant to take the complaint to the Healthcare Commission for an 'independent review'. The response should be signed by the primary care practitioner or the chief executive of the NHS body. If necessary, following investigation and with the agreement of the complainant, arrangements for conciliation or mediation should be made.

If a complainant is not happy with the results of 'local resolution' he or she may request the Healthcare Commission to undertake an independent review, and this also applies to complaints made to a foundation trust. The Healthcare Commission has ten working days to acknowledge receipt of the request.[25] It may decide to take no further action, to make recommendations to the NHS organisation concerned, to investigate further, to refer the complaint for consideration by a panel of lay persons, or in the case of foundation trusts, to Monitor; or to refer the complaint to a regulatory body such as the General Medical Council. The Commission's subsequent report, made to the complainant and the relevant NHS body or practitioner 'as soon as reasonably practical', should recommend any action required to resolve the problem and where appropriate make suggestions for improving the service in question. It should also detail the right of the complainant to take the complaint to the Health Service Ombudsman.

The Health Service Ombudsman

The Office of the Health Service Ombudsman is not part of the NHS. Also independent of the government, the Ombudsman provides independent consideration of complaints made by or on behalf of people who consider they have suffered due to unsatisfactory treatment by foundation trusts or to NHS services provided by the independent sector, as well as those provided by NHS trusts or primary care practitioners. The Ombudsman's remit encompasses unsatisfactory care, poor administration (such as misleading advice or mistakes over appointments), and failure to provide a service that should have been provided.

The Ombudsman will consider whether to investigate complaints made within a year of the event (or longer if the local investigation took longer than it should have done). The subsequent report is sent to the complainant, the organisation or practitioner involved, and the Secretary of State for Health. If a complaint is found to be justified the organisation or practitioner involved is 'asked' to provide a suitable remedy, other than financial compensation. There is no appeal from the findings of the Ombudsman.

Clinical negligence

The financial compensation of patients harmed through medical negligence (now commonly referred to as clinical negligence) is addressed through the legal system, with or without the involvement of the courts. Negligence claims are essentially disputes over acts or omissions which are alleged to have caused harm, and deal with who should pay compensation damages; the aim is, as far as possible, to put the claimant back in the position they would have been in had the act or omission not occurred. Under this system the claimant must prove the existence of a duty of care, that a breach of duty (i.e. negligence) occurred, that the negligence caused or was a material contribution to injury or damage, and the extent of the injury or damage.

Most primary care practitioners (GPs and dentists) and doctors working in private practice subscribe to a medical defence organisation, to provide them with legal and financial support in the event of a claim. Doctors working for NHS bodies, however, have been covered since the 1990s by the system of NHS Indemnity. Under this system NHS trusts, as the employers, are responsible for any legal and compensation costs of negligence claims against their doctors.

The NHS Litigation Authority

Since 1995 legal claims have been managed on behalf of the NHS by the NHS Litigation Authority, a special health authority (described in Chapter 2, pages 25–7) which runs a number of 'risk-pooling' schemes to spread the costs of medical negligence claims across the NHS as a whole. Although the number of claims per head of population is lower in England than in some other countries such as Sweden or New Zealand, the amounts paid per claim are much higher.[26] In 2003–4 the Litigation Authority received 6,251 claims of clinical negligence and 3,819 claims of non-clinical negligence against NHS bodies. In the same year £423 million was paid out in connection with clinical negligence claims, including both the damages paid to patients and the legal costs borne by the NHS. In 2004 total liabilities (the theoretical cost of paying all outstanding claims immediately, including those which had occurred but had not yet been formally reported), were estimated at £7.78 billion for clinical claims and £100 million for non-clinical claims.[27]

In 2003 the DH laid out proposals for a new system in the publication *Making Amends: A consultation paper setting out proposals for reforming the approach to clinical negligence in the NHS.* Providing an alternative to claims through the courts is intended to help deal with the rising costs of clinical negligence in the NHS. It involves an 'NHS Redress Scheme', to be run by the NHS Litigation Authority. It is composed of four main elements: an investigation of the incident and of any harm that has resulted; an explanation (to the patient) of the incident and of proposed action to prevent it recurring; the delivery of a package of remedial treatment and arrangements for continuing care when needed; and compensation payments for pain, suffering and out of pocket expenses, as well as for any needed care or treatment that the NHS cannot provide. Those accepting packages of care and compensation would be required to waive their rights to claim through the courts. The scheme was originally proposed with respect to hospital and community health services, but with the possibility of extending it to primary care services, and to NHS services provided by independent (private and voluntary) providers.

7   Research and development, and research governance

The Department of Health (DH) is the largest non-commercial funder of medical research in England. In 2005–6 the DH spent over £650 million on health-related research in England[1] via its NHS Research and Development (R&D) Programme and Policy Research Programme. In spring 2000 it published its strategy for the reform of funding and organisation of NHS R&D,[2] together with a research governance framework.[3] These announcements signalled an increased role for industry in NHS R&D, including identifying strategic objectives, setting priorities and delivering and exploiting clinical research. The reforms are designed to bring NHS research into line with the government's wider objectives of a mixed economy of provision in all aspects of health care and research.

This chapter shows how NHS R&D policy is now closely aligned with the rest of NHS policy. It begins by charting the development of NHS R&D policy from its inception, following a House of Lords report in 1988, through the 1990s and the creation of identifiable DH budgets for clinical research. It goes on to describe the latest reforms of R&D policy that have accompanied publication of *The NHS Plan*.

Research and development policy in the 1990s

In order to understand the most recent reforms of NHS R&D it is necessary to look back at the development of NHS R&D policy during the 1990s. The 1988 report of the Science and Technology Committee of the House of Lords identified a series of failings in the organisation and management of clinical research. The committee held that DH funding was needed to support research that would not be done if industry were the only producer of clinical research.[4]

As a result of the Committee's report an R&D programme was established within the DH under a Director of R&D, with a supporting structure in the form of the Clinical Research and Development Committee or CRDC. In 1991 the first director of R&D, Michael Peckham, made his first policy statement in the publication, *Research for Health: A Research and Development Strategy for the NHS*. The statement argued for a national programme of work on healthcare problems identified by the NHS, especially on the issues identified in the government's 1991 document, *The Health of the Nation*.

The internal market and the Culyer reforms

It was recognised that in order to deliver such a policy the DH would have to be able to quantify research activity throughout the NHS and to influence the way resources were devoted to it. The creation of an identifiable budget for research within the DH required a substantial reform of NHS finances. The real impetus behind financial reform, however, came from wider changes in NHS policy that were occurring in the early 1990s, in particular the likely impact of the 1990 NHS and Community Care Act, which created the internal market. This was seen by many as a serious threat to 'research-active' NHS trusts, which risked becoming uncompetitive, high-cost providers in the market for health care by virtue of their research activities. In response to these concerns a taskforce led by Professor Anthony Culyer was established in late 1993 with the aim of determining whether changes were needed in the organisation of, and support for, NHS R&D, and to advise on alternative funding and support mechanisms for it.

The Culyer taskforce reported in 1994.[5] It proposed changes in the mechanisms for deciding what R&D should be supported by the NHS, in the funding mechanisms themselves, and in accounting for NHS-funded R&D activity. The main recommendations are indicated in Box 7.1.

Prior to the Culyer reforms the costs of R&D were not identified and were met out of patient care budgets and through special allowances, such as a specific subvention for special health authorities, and a Service Increment for Teaching and Research, or SIFT, for undergraduate teaching hospitals. Crucially, the Culyer taskforce recommended that all monies previously spent on R&D be simplified and aggregated into a single national budget to which all the then health authorities would contribute. The national R&D budget became known as the 'NHS R&D Levy'. By 1997, the process had been refined and the new financial system fully implemented. Two streams of funding were financed from the R&D levy (see Box 7.2).

The first stream of R&D support funding was designed to provide service support to those NHS organisations involved in clinical research. 'Portfolio funding' was intended for the larger NHS trusts that could absorb all but major fluctuations in research activity as projects and programmes stop and start. 'Task-linked' funding was designed to be more responsive than portfolio funding and was aimed at NHS trusts, such as those with less research activity, which were less able to absorb changes in costs as new R&D activity began in their organisations.

The second stream of R&D funding was used to fund centrally-commissioned programmes of work which reflected national priorities.

Evaluating the Culyer reforms

There have been several reviews of NHS R&D under the Culyer reforms.[6] Most commentators agree that the reforms succeeded in helping to quantify the amount of money the NHS spends on R&D activity and brought about a more visible NHS R&D portfolio. The reforms also led to the development of R&D

Box 7.1   The main Culyer recommendations for NHS research and development (R&D)

- The real costs of R&D and patient care should be separated out, protecting NHS R&D from the potentially harmful effects of market conflict
- R&D funding should be allocated in a system of managed open competition, with R&D providers required to justify their claim on resources and be accountable for the R&D they do
- The new system should put all NHS providers, including the primary and community care sectors, on an equal footing with the acute sector in terms of access to funding for R&D and associated service costs

Source: Culyer, A., *Supporting Research and Development in the NHS*, 1994.

Box 7.2   Funding streams created under the Culyer reforms

R&D Support Funding for Providers ('Budget 1')

- Portfolio funding
- Task-linked funding

Centrally-managed NHS R&D programme ('Budget 2')

---

management functions within NHS organisations. They resulted in only a minimal redistribution of funding to primary care,[7] but as we have seen the main concern of the Culyer reforms was to protect the large teaching hospitals from the threat of disruption caused by the internal market, and in that they were successful. In 2005–6 more than 80 per cent of NHS spending on research – some £500 million – still occurred within the large hospital trusts, over two-thirds of it in London, mainly in the teaching hospitals.[8]

The extent to which the DH could influence the strategic direction of research, however, and manage research funding in line with its central objectives, remained limited. It is true that the national R&D programme enabled the DH to target funds at areas of national priority such as cancer, cardiovascular disease, strokes, mental health and the primary/secondary care interface, but these funds constituted only 5 per cent of the total. Most DH research funding was used to support bilateral agreements and concordats with the research councils (notably the Medical Research Council or MRC), the Higher Education Funding Council for England (HEFCE) and the large medical research charities, as well as supporting otherwise unfunded or 'own-account' research activity within the 'research active' NHS trusts. In practice the NHS did not exert control over the strategic direction of research council and charitable research funds; project- and programme-level decisions were made by the recipient funding organisations.

A strategic review of the R&D levy was commissioned by the Central Research and Development Committee or CRDC in 1997, and reported in 1999.[8] The review concluded that further changes were needed. Among the recommendations were a clearer focus on NHS needs and priorities, improved quality assurance systems, and greater involvement of wider healthcare communities and consumers in NHS R&D.

Research and development policy since 2000

In 2000 the DH published *Research and Development for a First Class Service: R&D funding in the New NHS,* in which it announced its plans to align clinical research more closely to the wider objectives of the NHS as set out in *The NHS Plan.* In line with recent changes in clinical services, the direction of change in NHS R&D has subsequently been towards public–private partnerships in setting strategic objectives, identifying priorities and delivering R&D.

The R&D strategy draws heavily on the strong, wider government initiative to increase the outputs from public sector research. An influential report entitled *Creating Knowledge Creating Wealth: Realising the Economic Potential of Public Sector Research Establishments* (the Baker Report), published by the Treasury in August 1999, set out the government's objectives for the commercialisation of public sector research. The report emphasised the government's policy of 'selling services into wider markets' and the need for research establishments to ensure that they identify the commercial potential of research and secure the effective transfer of knowledge to the private sector.[9] It was followed by the Department of Trade and Industry's white paper on science and innovation, *Excellence and Opportunity,* and the DH's response in its 2001 publication *Science and Innovation Strategy,* which mapped out a broader approach to the development of NHS R&D strategy and delivery. Central to this approach were changes in R&D funding streams, a new regulatory framework, changes to research ethics committees and the development of new collaborations, partnerships and networks.

Changes in funding

The aim of *Research & Development for a First Class Service* was to provide a clearer strategic direction for R&D activity by overhauling the existing funding streams and budgets. The DH subsequently published three supporting documents providing more details of the overhaul of funding streams.[10] At least notionally, the 'service support' funding element of the Culyer funding streams was replaced by two new streams: NHS Priorities and Needs Funding, or PNF, and support for science funding (see Box 7.3).

As with the funding budgets created under the Culyer reforms, the new funding streams could not be implemented immediately. The DH had hoped to allocate NHS support for science to hospital trusts on the basis of a national standard

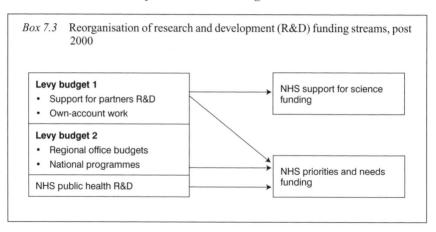

Box 7.3   Reorganisation of research and development (R&D) funding streams, post 2000

funding formula. Work on a standard formula began in May 2000 but by 2002, owing to the difficulties experienced in accessing data to underpin the formula, the DH opted for a much simpler, if cruder, approach. At least for the time being hospital trusts simply make annual declarations of the proportions of their R&D funding budgets that fall within the two new funding streams (priorities and needs funding and support for science funding).

Priorities and needs funding

NHS priorities and needs funding or PNF is intended to support priorities set out in the national service frameworks or NSFs (see Chapter 6, page 114) and the work of the National Institute for Health and Clinical Excellence (NICE, described in Chapter 6, page 113–4). It is also designed to support R&D in public health and epidemiology, primary care and health services. In order to receive priorities and needs funding NHS organisations must be able to show that they are working in collaborative research partnerships with other NHS trusts, PCTs, universities or other partners. In England three programmes, commissioned nationally, were also established within PNF: service delivery and organisation (SDO), health technology assessment (HTA), and new and emerging applications of technology (NEAT).

Support for science funding

NHS support for science funding is designed to provide hospital trusts with an income stream that enables them to meet the service support costs incurred by R&D activity that is funded by the research councils (e.g. the Medical Research Council) and other eligible R&D funding partners, such as medical research charities, whose research grants do not cover such costs. The principles of support for science funding are largely the same as those of the Culyer funding levy discussed on page 137 above, i.e. to provide financial stability for large NHS trusts.

A research governance framework

A further key objective of the DH's science and innovation policy is 'to ensure that the rights, health, and safety of the public and patients are protected and their interests reflected.'[11] Central to this objective is the introduction of a new regulatory framework for research related to health and social care, as outlined in the 2001 publication, *Research Governance Framework for Health and Social Care*. The framework is intended to make it possible to manage the risks arising from health research, and is an attempt to ensure compliance with the relevant professional, ethical and legal standards that impinge on clinical research. Increasingly, these standards are enshrined in law. For instance, as well as the requirement to ensure compliance with legal frameworks such as the Data Protection Act (1998), the Human Rights Act (1998), and the Health and Safety at Work Act (1974), research-active organisations must also take steps to ensure compliance with new sets of legal regulations such as the EU Clinical Trials Directive, and others made under the Human Tissue Act and the Mental Capacity Act.

Research governance is now one of the Healthcare Standards with which PCTs as well as hospital trusts must comply, and they must give evidence of how the standard is being met. Most aspects of the research governance framework are, however, mainly the concern of NHS trusts, which must have in place the internal structures needed to enable new research policies and procedures to be developed, and research conduct to be adequately overseen. This means that research-active NHS organisations are now much more involved in monitoring and auditing research projects, as well as providing relevant training and education programmes for their staff. The support funding allocations to NHS trusts, however, which were set at the time of the Culyer reforms, have not been significantly increased to support NHS trusts in the task of ensuring compliance with the new regulations (although in early 2005 the DH did announce a small increase in funding allocations to help defray the costs of the EU Clinical Trials Directive).

The research governance framework identifies the many stakeholders in clinical research and defines their responsibilities. Central to the framework is the concept of 'research sponsor', one organisation that is responsible for ensuring that the design of the study meets appropriate standards and that arrangements are in place to ensure appropriate conduct and reporting. The concept of sponsor is not new in commercial research, where the pharmaceutical industry has traditionally had to meet the requirements of regional and national regulatory offices in order to obtain the necessary marketing authorisations for new products undergoing their first use in humans. The requirement for a legally accountable sponsor is new for non-commercial trials, which are often managed informally through collaborative agreements between NHS trusts, universities and trials units. Most non-commercial trials are lower-risk, in that they involve the testing of long-marketed products in new indications or in combination with other products. At the time of writing it remains unclear how the regulatory offices – the Medicines

and Healthcare Products Regulatory Agency (MHRA),* in the case of the UK
– will expect sponsorship to be implemented for non-commercial clinical trials,
where the concept of a sole sponsor does not fit readily.[12]

Research ethics committees

Alongside the implementation of the research governance framework, significant
changes have been introduced in the way research ethics committees operate, and
in their accountability arrangements. Traditionally research ethics committees
have been part of the self-governing arrangements of the medical profession,
responsible for scientific quality and safety and for ensuring that the risks of
research have been adequately communicated to patients or others taking part in
research trials. To ensure compliance with the EU clinical trials directive, research
ethics committees are now being drawn into a new centralised structure overseen
by a Central Office for Research Ethics Committees or COREC, part of the
National Patient Safety Agency (see Chapter 6, page 126). As safety and scientific
quality will be the responsibility of the research sponsor or host organisation for
the research, the emphasis in an ethics committee review will be to ensure that
the risks of research have been adequately communicated to patients or others
taking part in research trials, and ethics committees will perhaps have reduced
responsibilities. A review of the ethics committee reforms is being undertaken,
in a context of growing unrest within the clinical academic community about
increasingly bureaucratic research review procedures.[13]

New collaborations, partnerships and networks in clinical research

Various changes in clinical R&D have been initiated to 'form a platform to bring
in other players from industry and the science base on a collaborative basis to
maximise opportunities for innovation and research'.[11] This strategy is perhaps
most visible in the Pharmaceutical Industry Competitiveness Taskforce or PICTF,
a partnership between industry and the government. This was established in
April 2000, largely in response to industry concerns about threats to the UK's
competitiveness in pharmaceutical research. Although its remit was not restricted
to an examination of the factors that influence the competitiveness of the clinical
research environment in the UK, it is leading to a reshaping of that environment.
The taskforce saw three factors as central: speed (in terms of the start-up times of
clinical research), quality and cost. A focus on these factors is central to the work
of the new collaborations, partnerships and networks, outlined below, which have
been established to set strategic objectives, identify priorities and facilitate and
fund research in the government's priority areas.

---

*   The MHRA is taking on an inspection function for all non-commercial and probably
    some commercial research. This will eventually be funded through a 'full cost recovery'
    system, charging organisations the full cost of inspecting research programmes or
    studies.

Cancer research networks

Cancer was identified by the DH as one of its first priority areas and it is in this area that the network model of setting strategy and R&D delivery is the most developed. Following the publication of a report on cancer research by the House of Commons Science and Technology Committee,[14] and the publication of the *National Cancer Plan*, a National Cancer Research Institute (NCRI) was established in April 2001 to plan and co-ordinate cancer research across the UK. The Institute was set up as a partnership between the government, the voluntary sector and the private sector, and published its first strategic report in October 2002.[15] The report discussed the current levels of cancer research activity across England and identified issues which would benefit from a more sustained research effort. Attempts to develop a more co-ordinated strategic approach to cancer research involving all funders are also evident in the establishment of a Cancer Research Funders Forum or CRFF, whose membership includes all the major cancer research funding bodies.

Supporting the National Cancer Research Institute are two networks which are taking forward the new strategic objectives. First, a National Cancer Research Network or NCRN has been established, with a budget of £20 million, to provide the necessary infrastructure and to ensure increased patient recruitment to cancer clinical trials. To meet its aims, the National Network has established local cancer research networks covering the same areas as the 34 cancer service networks across England. London alone has five such networks, each with a budget of up to £500,000 a year. The National Network also operates a trial 'adoption' scheme which enables researchers to tap into the additional resources and support available through the network, but does not take any of the research governance and sponsorship requirements away from the NHS trusts that are hosting the research.

Secondly, a National Translational Cancer Research Network or NTRAC has been established to ensure that new scientific discoveries in cancer therapy can be translated quickly from the laboratory to routine clinical treatment. A network of ten centres has emerged, based on centres of academic and clinical excellence, each receiving £1 million over five years to build infrastructure and workforce capability. In addition to these activities the Translational Network is establishing a national tumour tissue bank of tissue collected from patients for commercial and academic use. There is also evidence that the Translational Network is putting pressure on hospital trusts to standardise research costs and drive them down, thereby contributing to the more favourable 'platform' for industry that is emphasised in the DH's Science and Innovation Strategy.[11]

Other clinical research networks

Mental health was the second government priority area to adopt a network model for research strategy and delivery. The network, which consists of eight regional networks across England, aims to make possible large-scale, multi-centre, multi-disciplinary research studies in mental health. Like the National Cancer Research

Network it plays an increasingly important role in determining which research gets the go-ahead.

Two reports have done much to contribute to the growth of the partnership and network model in clinical R&D strategy and delivery. *Bioscience 2015: Improving National Health, Increasing National Wealth* was published in 2003 by the Bioscience Innovation and Growth Team. This team was established by the Department of Trade and Industry in late 2002 with a remit to identify barriers holding back the growth of the bioscience industry in the UK, and to recommend ways to enhance the competitiveness of the UK bioscience industry. Its report recommended collaboration between the NHS and industry, the creation of a supportive regulatory environment, greater investments in biomedical R&D and the use of the NHS to speed up the approval and acceptance of 'breakthrough' treatments.

Similar recommendations were made in a 2003 report published by the Academy of Medical Sciences called *Strengthening Clinical Research*. This report highlighted the 'substantial gulf between basic discoveries and converting such discoveries into innovations that directly benefit patients or prevent disease'.[16] It listed several key reasons, including inappropriate facilities and infrastructure, lack of clinical scientists, inadequate funding, an increasingly complex regulatory environment and the failure to utilise fully the opportunity offered by the NHS for clinical research.

In response to these two reports the DH established a Research for Patient Benefit Working Party in 2003, to propose how their recommendations should be taken forward. The working party reported in 2004 and recommended principally the creation of a UK Clinical Research Collaboration to 'establish the NHS as the world leader in contributions to clinical research' and to achieve this through the 'power of partnership'.[17] The Collaboration is a partnership between government, the voluntary sector, industry and patients. The working party also recommended the creation of a UK Clinical Research Network, a co-ordinating body for more research networks focusing specifically on specific diseases or groups of diseases on the lines of the existing cancer and mental health networks. Initial priority has been given to medicines for children, Alzheimer's disease, stroke and diabetes. At the time of writing the new networks are still under development.

Non-disease-specific networks

Crucial to the government's strategy concerning NHS intellectual property is the opening up of several Department of Trade and Industry funding streams to enable NHS trusts to build capacity and support the creation of networks for the management and commercial exploitation of their intellectual property. As well as the Department of Trade and Industry Biotechnology Exploitation Platform scheme, a fund from which NHS trusts can now bid for financial support, a £10 million Public Sector Research Establishment fund has been established 'to enable public sector bodies carrying out research to have access to the skills and expertise needed to evaluate the commercial potential of their work and to take steps to bring ideas towards exploitation.'[18] In line with the recommendations of the already-mentioned Baker Report, *Creating knowledge creating wealth,* which called for the creation of networks for commercialising public-sector research, twelve intellectual property 'hubs', consisting of networks of hospital trusts and PCTs, have been established to provide a structure of support and expertise.

The intellectual property hubs will eventually exist as external, publicly-owned or joint-venture commercial organisations, with which NHS organisations will make contracts. To this end the hubs will take advantage of new legislation which supports the strategy of moving towards public–private partnerships in NHS R&D by enabling NHS organisations to form spin-off companies. Section 5 of the Health and Social Care Act (2001) gives NHS organisations freedom to work with external investors in developing and marketing their intellectual property. NHS trusts and their employees will be able to take a shareholding in spin-off companies created specifically to take commercial advantage of intellectual property generated by their research programmes.

Other new public–private partnerships

There are numerous other examples of public–private co-operation in clinical R&D. For instance funding from the Department of Trade and Industry has been used to establish five Genetics Knowledge Parks across England. The aim is for the knowledge parks to contribute to emerging developments in genetics, from the development of test methods to evaluating the requirement for counselling patients. The emerging strategy for genetics research brings together the NHS R&D science base, industry and the charitable sector.

Department of Trade and Industry funding has also been used to support the initiation of the Medical Devices Faraday Partnership, which includes six UK universities and several major UK companies. The partnership aims to shorten the time taken to get new products to market and generate new business opportunities for UK healthcare companies. At the time of writing it remains unclear how the partnership will relate to the NHS, or how improvements in patient care arising from its work will be managed.

New strategy for clinical research and development

In the summer of 2005 the DH went out to consultation on perhaps its most radical strategic plan for NHS R&D to date. Central to the strategy is the creation of a new National Institute for Health Research which it is hoped will give UK clinical research a higher international profile. There are also proposals to create up to 10 Academic Medical Centres (AMCs), or 'premier research hospitals'. £100 million are being made available over four years to enable the creation of the AMCs, which the DH hopes to see developing strong international reputations akin to those of the Mayo clinics and Massachusetts General clinics in the USA, and the EU's 'centres of excellence'. The strategy, entitled *Best Research for Best Health: A New National Health Research Strategy,* lays fresh emphasis on the network approach to NHS R&D strategy, delivery and governance, and a further overhaul of R&D funding streams is also planned.[19]

An important part of the new strategy is the creation of more Clinical Research Facilities (CRFs), five of which are already in existence across England and Scotland. The CRFs, which focus on experimental medicine and aim to speed up the translation of scientific advances into the clinic, are Wellcome Trust initiatives in collaboration with the Wolfson Foundation and the Departments of Health in England, Scotland, Wales and Northern Ireland.

Conclusion

There are many parallels between NHS R&D strategy and recent developments in the funding and delivery of NHS services. There is an increasing emphasis on public–private partnerships, both in the provision of health services and in R&D, and new funding streams, collaborations, partnerships and networks are being put into place to support this. The new partnerships and networks have the potential to add much-needed strategic direction to NHS R&D activity, which was largely missing during the 1990s. But the potential for conflicts of interest is significant as the new partnerships and networks pave the way for industry to take on a much greater role in influencing the strategic direction and delivery of NHS R&D. As Harrison and New point out, the attempts to improve the public–private interface in clinical R&D 'are largely designed to support the role of the private rather than the public sector.'[20] The extent to which the NHS's duty of care may be compromised by financial or other incentives is particularly sensitive.

The research governance framework has also been put in place largely to oversee the transition to a mixed economy of R&D provision. It will potentially enhance the protection of research subjects through a sharing of responsibility between the medical profession, academic and healthcare organisations and the law, and by increased public involvement. Its effectiveness depends, however, on the degree of clarity it brings to the roles and responsibilities of all the stakeholders in research, and the extent to which the objectives of industry, the NHS and the public can be effectively conflated.

8   The NHS workforce

In September 2004 the NHS employed 1.3 million people,[1] making it the largest employer in Europe. Although clinical staff constitute the largest group, due to the large number of nursing staff, the largest growth since 1997 has been in managerial staff, with a 70 per cent increase in numbers (see Table 8.1).

Expansion of the workforce has been central to the government's plans for the modernisation of the NHS; increased staff numbers are recognised to be essential for achieving greater capacity in order to address waiting list targets, and to achieve the reduction in junior doctors' working hours required by the European Working Time Directive. National targets for expansion were laid out in *The NHS Plan* and subsequently updated in the 2003–6 priorities and planning framework.*[2] But as responsibility for service provision has been devolved to 'frontline' organisations, so too has responsibility for workforce planning; the DH is now 'moving away from an emphasis on centrally prescribed national targets on doctor and nurse numbers to a reliance on credible local plans that maximise workforce capacity to support delivery.'[3] Thus workforce development is now an important part of the local planning function: PCTs, working with provider organisations (NHS trusts, foundation trusts and independent sector providers), now undertake workforce planning as part of their local delivery plans. This is overseen by the Strategic Health Authority (SHA) for their area, which aggregates local delivery plans to produce 'capacity plans'. Representatives of SHAs meet as the National Workforce Group, to inform and influence policy and practice in workforce planning.

An increased NHS workforce is to be achieved by creating more training places for new nursing staff and therapists, and more places in medical schools, and by re-structuring post-graduate medical education to shorten the time taken to become a consultant. At the same time there has been an emphasis on staff 'working differently', allowing non-medical practitioners to take on functions previously undertaken by doctors. This change includes giving prescribing rights to nurses and pharmacists, the development of 'nurse consultants' and 'emergency care practitioners', and the development of GPs with special interests to take over

---

*   The updated targets were for an extra 15,000 doctors, 35,000 nurses and 30,000 therapists and scientists by 2008, from a 2001 baseline.

Table 8.1   Numbers of NHS staff (headcount), 1997 to 2004

	1997	2004	Change (%)
Consultants	21,474	30,650	43
Non-consultant hospital doctors	30,313	41,697	38
GPs	29,389	34,085	16
Nurses, midwives and health visitors	300,467	375,371	25
Nurses working in General Practice	18,389	22,144	20
Professions allied to medicine	45,022	58,959	31
Other therapeutic, scientific and ambulance staff	66,217	87,196	32
Support to clinical staff	283,871	368,285	30
Managerial staff	22,173	37,726	70
Central functions	70,647	99,831	41
Hotel, property and estates	77,803	73,932	− 5
'Other'	92,921	101,211	9
Total	1,058,686	1,331,087	26

Source: Department of Health, *All Staff in the NHS, 1994–2004*. London, 2005.

various functions, such as outpatient endoscopy, that have hitherto been performed in hospitals.

Other countries are also considered an important source of trained staff. Recruitment in countries such as the Philippines, South Africa, and India has meant that in the year to March 2003 there were over 13,000 overseas entrants on the nursing register who intended to work in the UK.[4] The government also began an international advertising campaign for GPs and hospital consultants in 2001, and in 2002 launched an NHS international fellowship scheme to offer two-year fellowships to experienced surgeons and physicians from outside the UK to work as consultants in the NHS. Between 1999 and 2004 the number of hospital doctors who had qualified outside the UK rose from 19,689 (31 per cent) to 29,974 (37 per cent). Most of these (25,238, or 31 per cent of all hospital doctors) qualified outside the European Economic Area. Most are in non-consultant grades; concentrated in the 'staff grades' and 'associate specialist' groups,* they account for over 60 per cent of the doctors in these categories.[5] The use of corporate providers from overseas is also seen as a source of additional staff.

Medical staff

Doctors or 'medical staff' make up 9 per cent of the total NHS workforce. The 106,432 doctors working for the NHS comprise 72,347 hospital doctors and 34,085 GPs (Table 8.1). With only 2.2 practising physicians per 1,000 population,[6] the UK has one of the lowest ratios of doctors per head in Europe (Table 8.2).

Doctors achieve their basic medical qualification in university medical schools, with attachments in affiliated hospitals providing clinical experience. The degree course has traditionally taken five years, although a shorter four-year degree course has now been introduced for mature students and graduates in other fields. Once qualified, doctors are required to work for a year in a recognised training position before they can achieve full registration with the General Medical Council. A move to 'modernise medical careers', begun in 2003, has changed the post-graduate training of doctors, which although structured was strongly dependent on learning from experience. The new system of training is intended to be a more structured and formal approach, to streamline doctors' career paths and shorten the time they take to achieve accreditation in their chosen specialties. On leaving medical school doctors now work in a two-year 'foundation programme' which provides experience and 'tasters' in a broad range of specialties. They then enter training programmes within their chosen specialties, and on completion are awarded a certificate of completion of training, or CCT, to become accredited as either a GP or a hospital specialist (or

---

* Staff grades and associate specialist grades are non-training positions, which do not offer progression to consultant status but which are needed in order to fulfil service commitments.

Table 8.2   Doctors per 1,000 population, 2003, by country

Country	Doctors per 1,000 population
United Kingdom	2.2
United States	2.3
Sweden	3.3
France	3.4
Germany	3.4
Italy	4.1

Source: Organisation for Economic Co-operation and Development, health data 2005 – country notes.

'consultant'), eligible to be entered onto the General Medical Council's specialist register. At the time of writing it seems likely that, at least for the medical specialties, elements of general and specialist training and accreditation will be separated out. Doctors will be able to undertake shorter training programmes in general medicine, become accredited as consultants in general medicine or surgery to work in hospitals and provide general medical care such as for emergency admissions, and then subsequently be able to train in a specialist area, such as cardiology or urology, to become further accredited in that field.

The post-graduate training and education of doctors is overseen by a recently-established Postgraduate Medical Education and Training Board (PMETB), a non-executive departmental public body described in Chapter 2 (page 34). It has UK-wide responsibility for developing and approving programmes of training, setting entry standards, approving curricula, and recruiting, developing and assessing educational supervisors. It also sets the standards for the completion of specialist training, issues certificates of completion of training (CCTs), and makes recommendations on applications for entry to the GMC's register of accredited specialists. Some of these roles were previously performed by the Royal Medical Colleges, which comprise many of the hospital-based medical specialties as well as general practice. Hitherto the Royal Colleges have played a central role in the education and training of doctors, providing education and training courses, setting educational standards, setting and running post-graduate exams, and approving training posts in hospitals. The Colleges remain involved in all this in the appointment process for senior (consultant) positions, both in approving positions as appropriate for consultant status, and in interviewing candidates for consultant posts;* and continue to collaborate with the PMETB in policy-making for medical education and training. But the leading role has passed to the PMETB.

Limits on the number of training positions within specialist training schemes have resulted in a shortage of middle-grade doctors available to fill the service commitments of NHS hospitals. This shortfall is increasingly being filled by doctors working in a variety of non-training posts which have been invented by hospital trusts to fill their service gaps. They are often personal appointments for doctors who for various reasons have been unable to undertake or complete higher specialist training in a hospital specialty. Known as 'non-consultant career grades' they include 'staff grades', consisting of doctors who tend to work alongside junior doctors in training positions, and at a more senior level, 'associate specialists'. Associate specialists tend to be doctors who are close to consultants in their level of experience and often perform similar duties, but are technically accountable to a consultant. There is also a category known as 'clinical assistants', usually local

---

* Unlike NHS trusts, FTs are not obliged to involve the Royal Colleges in the appointment of medical staff. In 2005, however, a concordat was signed between the foundation trust 'network', a body which represents all current foundation trusts, and the Royal Colleges, enabling the organisations to work together on the appointment of consultant medical staff for FTs.

GPs who work a fixed number of sessions in a hospital speciality, such as accident and emergency.

Doctors working in the hospital sector hold contracts of employment with their hospital trusts but work on nationally-agreed terms and conditions of service. They have traditionally been salaried, although a sort of 'fee for service' scheme was piloted in a number of NHS trusts in 2004–5, whereby consultants received bonus payments for performing extra work. In contrast most GPs are self-employed independent practitioners (see Chapter 4, pages 50–1), working in partnerships and operating as small businesses, the partners often owning their own premises and employing their own staff. These partnerships, rather than individual GPs, hold the contracts with their local PCTs to provide services. The contracts are mostly on national terms and conditions known as General Medical Services or GMS arrangements, but increasingly under locally-negotiated terms and conditions known as Personal Medical Services or PMS. As discussed in Chapter 4 (page 52), by 2004 almost 40 per cent of GPs were working under PMS arrangements.[7] Under both GMS and PMS arrangements a significant minority of GPs – 9 per cent in 2004[8] – choose to work on salaried terms, receiving salaries for working an agreed number of clinical sessions.

A number of other independent practitioners also provide general medical services for the NHS, under contracts held with PCTs. They include some 19,300 dentists,[9] 8,331 opthalmic practitioners,[10] and pharmacists working in some 10,000 pharmacies.[11] Achieving their primary qualifications through university degree courses they then operate as independent practitioners, either setting up their own businesses or working for an established business or corporation. NHS work is undertaken on a contract basis, the practice (rather than the practitioner) being remunerated according to a national schedule.

Nursing staff

Nurses, health visitors and midwives form the largest group of NHS clinical staff; the 375,371 working in the NHS in 2004 comprise 28 per cent of the NHS workforce (Table 8.1). Of the total 7 per cent were midwives, 3 per cent district nurses and 4 per cent health visitors.[12] The UK Nursing and Midwifery Council (NMC) oversees their training and registration and holds a register of all those eligible to practise. Nurses and midwives undertake their training within institutes of higher education to either diploma or degree level, combining theory and supervised nursing practice. Some NHS trusts also offer 'cadet schemes', intended to offer a route into nursing for local people between the ages of 16 and 19. A form of modern apprenticeship, these schemes provide placements in hospital settings such as wards, physiotherapy departments, and reception, offering practical experience as well as an opportunity to complete National Vocational Qualifications or a nursing access course.*

---

*   Healthcare assistants (also known as nursing auxiliaries) often work alongside nurses in both hospital and community settings to provide care such as washing and dressing

Nursing degree courses are longer than diploma courses (four years as opposed to three) but enable nurses to apply, later in their careers, for senior positions and positions in nurse education and management. Both nurses and midwives can undertake a further one-year degree-level course to become health visitors, responsible for the health of infants and young children in the community.

Extending the role of nurses was one of the key aims of *The NHS Plan*, and forms part of the government's intention to increase the capacity of the NHS workforce by increasing the number of staff 'working differently'. This has resulted in many nurses developing specialist skills, enabling them to manage a clinical case-load independently. With varying titles, such as 'clinical nurse specialists' or 'nurse practitioners', they can order tests and investigations, run clinics, perform minor surgical procedures and prescribe medications; they work in a variety of locations, from NHS trusts to NHS walk-in centres, primary and community care settings, and hospices. In 2001 the development of the nursing role was taken further with the creation of 'nurse consultant' posts. The role of nurse consultants is to improve the quality of health care provision and strengthen professional leadership; in addition to a clinical commitment of at least 50 per cent of their time they also play roles in leadership, education and training, practice and service development, and research and evaluation. By 2004 there were 631 nurse consultants in England.[12]

Allied health professionals

Allied health professionals form part of the multi-disciplinary teams providing care to patients. They often work one-to-one with patients and may have their own case-loads. Encompassing a broad range of disciplines they provide both clinical and technical services, including those of chiropodists/podiatrists, dieticians, occupational therapists, orthoptists*, physiotherapists, speech and language therapists, paramedics and ambulance staff, radiographers, prosthetists,† and drama art and music therapists. Taken together the 58,959 allied health professionals in the NHS constitute approximately 4 per cent of its workforce.[12]

The way in which allied health professionals are trained obviously varies; many, such as physiotherapists, radiographers and orthoptists, undertake three-year degree courses at universities which enable them to achieve state registration

---

patients, bed-making, toileting, and monitoring patients by, for example, measuring their weight, temperature, and blood pressures. They can obtain National Vocational Qualifications (NVQ) in care; the achievement of a level three NVQ makes them eligible for entry into nurse training.

* Orthoptists work in both hospitals and community settings, screening for visual defects in school children as well as diagnosing and treating defects of vision and abnormalities of eye movement (such as squints) in patients referred to them by GPs or hospital consultants.

† Prosthetists and orthotists provide care and equipment for anyone requiring an artificial limb (prosthesis) or a device to support or control part of the body, such as a brace or splint (orthosis). They also advise on rehabilitation.

and take positions in the NHS. Others, such as music and drama therapists, train via post-graduate diploma courses, typically of a year's duration, while ambulance technicians and paramedics are trained by ambulance trusts* through salaried posts, typically taking a year to achieve their qualifications.

In 2000 the DH publication *Meeting the Challenge: A Strategy for the Allied Health Professions* recognised their important contribution to improving patients' outcomes and experience. It introduced the concept of extended roles for allied health professionals, and declared the government's intention to create allied health professional consultants. These will work with greater autonomy and have leadership, education, training and research responsibilities, for example teaching staff from all healthcare disciplines and working with senior medical and nursing colleagues to help draw up local care and referral protocols.

Other staff

The NHS workforce also includes a vast range of non-clinical staff who provide infrastructure and support services. These include scientific and therapeutic staff, such as pharmacists, laboratory staff, and equipment technicians. They also include staff performing central functions such as personnel, finance, information technology, and legal services, and staff working in the 'hotel', property and estates services who provide maintenance, laundry, catering and gardening services. They also include managerial staff responsible for budgets, manpower, or assets, and staff who are accountable for significant areas of work.

While the number of staff providing central functions and managerial services has increased steadily since 1997, the number of staff providing support services such as hotel, property and estates services has declined (Table 8.1). This reflects the continuation of the 1980s' policy of 'out-sourcing' non-clinical services such as catering, laundry and cleaning to private sector companies. The trend has been further advanced by the transfer of many such staff to private sector employment when new hospitals are built under the Private Finance Initiative.

The way in which staff are trained for all these roles varies widely. For example pharmacists require a four-year degree-level qualification, followed by a year of practical training, before they can be state-registered and eligible to work in the NHS. Other scientific staff, such as laboratory assistants and equipment technicians, as well as many non-clinical support staff in the 'hotel' and estates services, are trained 'on the job'.

Entry into NHS management is by a number of routes. In-service management training is available to staff already employed in the NHS, through a programme leading to National Vocational Qualifications. A graduate training scheme exists to encourage the entry of graduates into areas such as general management, accountancy, and human resources, by providing a programme of work placements as well as the opportunity to gain post-graduate qualifications. There is also the 'NHS Gateway to Leadership Programme'. This recruits experienced managers

---

*   There are 31 ambulance trusts which provide ambulance services across England.

from a variety of organisations with the potential to progress to senior NHS management positions. Placements within senior management positions provide a 'fast track', whereby candidates are expected to become chief executives or directors of NHS trusts within five years.

Trade unions

Staff working in the health service are represented by several different unions. The largest is Unison, which has more than 400,000 members employed by the Health Service.[13] It is the major union representing both nursing and midwifery staff and administrative and clerical staff. Its membership also includes NHS staff in other groups such as allied health professionals, scientific and technical staff, and ancillary and maintenance staff such as cleaners and porters. AMICUS, with 80,000 members in the health sector,[14] represents staff from a wide range of non-medical occupations including nursing, midwifery and healthcare assistants, allied health professionals, and scientific, technical and dental staff, as well as administrative, clerical, ancillary and maintenance staff. The GMB also has some 30,000 members working in a wide range of non-medical healthcare fields,[15] while the Public and Commercial Services Union is one of several unions representing civil servants concerned with the NHS, and represents a substantial number of staff in the Department of Health. Doctors are mainly represented by the British Medical Association or BMA, with a total membership of over 134,000, including more than 3,000 from overseas.[16] Approximately 75 per cent of practising doctors in the UK are members.

9 Devolution: the NHS in Scotland, Wales and Northern Ireland

Since 1999 the NHS in Scotland, Wales and Northern Ireland has been organised and run separately from the NHS in England. Historical, constitutional and other factors had already led to some differences in health services organisation and policy between the four countries of the United Kingdom. Devolution has tended to make such differences more significant. This chapter provides a very brief overview of the structure and organisation of the NHS in Scotland, Wales and Northern Ireland.*

Funding

Despite political devolution the governments or 'executives' of Scotland, Wales and Northern Ireland remain dependent on the Westminster Parliament for funding. The 'devolved' countries have historically received more funding per head of population than England. Their allocations have been determined through negotiations between the Treasury and the former Scottish Office, Welsh Office, and Northern Ireland Office.[1] In Scotland the negotiations resulted in a formula known as the Barnett formula, with similar formulae for Wales and Northern Ireland. Since the 1970s, however, any increases in NHS funding have been distributed on the basis of the relative populations of the four countries of the UK. Over time this is intended to result in a gradual convergence of their per capita funding levels.

Responsibility for allocating resources to different services and different areas within each country lies with its parliament or assembly. Broadly speaking resources are distributed on the basis of healthcare need, using formulae based on population, adjusted for measures of healthcare need, such as age, sex and morbidity, and for the extra costs of providing services in rural or sparsely populated areas.

In Scotland the organisations providing services – hospitals, GPs, ambulance services, etc. – receive annual budgets. In Wales and Northern Ireland, however,

* Readers who need more detail should refer as a starting-point to the website of the NHS in the relevant country: NHS Scotland: http://www.show.scot.nhs.uk; NHS Wales: http://www.wales.nhs.uk ; NHS Northern Ireland: www.dhsspsni.gov.uk.

a 'purchaser–provider split', broadly similar to that in England, means that the organisations providing services receive their funding as 'income' received or 'earned' from organisations which commission or 'purchase' their services. However Wales and Northern Ireland have yet to introduce England's 'payment by results' system, (described in Chapter 5, pages 96–9).

Structures

The Scottish Parliament and the Welsh and Northern Ireland Assemblies have varying legislative powers with respect to health care, so that Westminster legislation affects them to varying degrees. Furthermore their governments, or executives, are individually responsible for developing health policy and overseeing the delivery of healthcare services, leading to further divergences.

Broadly speaking, since devolution Scotland has moved furthest away from the structure of the English NHS, especially by abolishing the 'purchaser–provider split' originally introduced in Scotland in the early 1990s as part of the internal market. The NHS in Scotland is now once again an integrated system, with a single body – the Scottish Department of Health – responsible for planning and providing all healthcare services. Use of the independent (private and voluntary) sectors by the NHS in Scotland has also been limited, resorted to in order to ease waiting lists rather than being viewed as a source of 'mainstream' providers of care, as in England. In contrast Wales has adopted a model more similar to England's: local bodies analogous to England's PCTs are responsible for overseeing the provision of primary care services and for commissioning or 'purchasing' hospital and community health services from NHS trusts. So far, however, Wales has not followed England in creating foundation trusts, or in commissioning more NHS care from the private sector. Northern Ireland has seen the least change in the organisation of its NHS, since devolution, and has a structure similar to that of the NHS internal market in England. Regional bodies and their sub-committees commission or 'purchase' the full range of healthcare services for their populations. On the other hand, in Northern Ireland, unlike all the other countries of the UK, it is the NHS, not local authorities, which provides social care services.

The NHS in Scotland

The NHS in Scotland (NHS Scotland) serves a population of around 5 million.[2] It has approximately 132,000 staff, the largest group being some 63,000 nurses, midwives and health visitors. There are some 8,500 doctors working in hospital and community health services, as well as more than 7,000 family practitioners (GPs, dentists, opticians and pharmacists) providing services under contract to the NHS.[3]

The NHS in Scotland was established in 1947 under a separate NHS (Scotland) Act, so that it has always operated as a separate entity from the NHS in England, with separate legislation needed for all major changes to the system. This autonomy was strengthened by political devolution in 1999. For 'devolved functions', which include health,* the Scottish Parliament can pass primary legislation and amend or repeal existing Acts of the UK Parliament.

In 2000 the Scottish government (the Scottish Executive) published its own version of the English NHS Plan, with the publication of *Our National Health: A Plan for Action, a Plan for Change*. This outlined its intention of moving away from the 'purchaser–provider split' introduced in the 1990s. A 2003 policy statement called *Partnerships for Care* outlined the intended structural reform, and legislation followed: the 2002 Community Care and Health (Scotland) Act, the 2004 Primary Medical Services (Scotland) Act, and the 2004 NHS Reform (Scotland) Act. Further policy proposals, *Building a Health Service Fit for the Future: A National Framework for Service Change in the NHS in Scotland* (the Kerr Report), were published in 2005.

The structure of the NHS in Scotland

With the abolition of the 'purchaser–provider' split, the structure of NHS Scotland is now the one shown in Figure 9.1.

Organisations with strategic roles

THE SCOTTISH EXECUTIVE AND ITS HEALTH DEPARTMENT

The Scottish Executive is responsible for developing health policy, for allocating healthcare resources and for delivering healthcare services, through 'NHS Scotland'. It performs these tasks through The Scottish Executive Health Department or SEHD, under a Minister for Health and Community Care. The SEHD performs its functions through five 'directorates': human resources (for the whole of NHS Scotland); nursing (which includes allied health professionals such as physiotherapists and radiographers); service delivery, policy and planning; performance management and finance (of NHS Scotland organisations); and health improvement (through preventative healthcare policies). These directorates are each further sub-divided into divisions. As in the English DH, professional advice is provided to the SEHD by a Chief Medical Officer and a Chief Nursing Officer.

The SEHD also has a 'national waiting times unit', overseeing initiatives aimed at reducing waiting times, such as the purchase of a private hospital (see below, page 158) or the use of the independent sector to provide elective services. The SEHD has also established a 'Centre for Change and Innovation' or CCI, intended to help implement service improvements in priority areas by spreading change and

---

* A number of health policy areas are 'retained' by Westminster and fall outside the jurisdiction of the Scottish Parliament. These include the regulation of healthcare professionals, abortion and human fertilisation issues, xenotransplantation, and the control and safety of medicines.

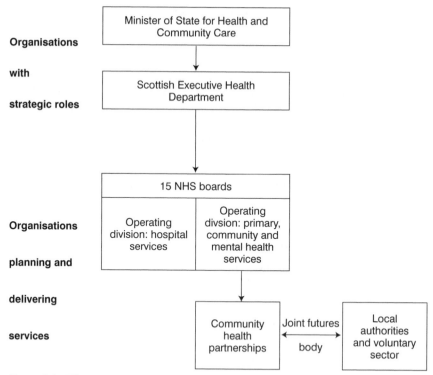

Figure 9.1   The structure of NHS Scotland

'best practice' throughout NHS Scotland organisations. It operates by supporting local 'service redesign committees' which are responsible for developing plans to redesign and modernise services in their area.

The SEHD has a number of 'arm's length bodies', which it funds to undertake various functions. There are seven 'special health boards', analogous to the special health authorities in England (see Chapter 2 pages 23–30):

1   NHS 24, a 24-hour telephone information and advice service.
2   NHS Education for Scotland (NES), a training organisation providing courses and educational programmes for NHS Scotland's staff.
3   NHS Health Scotland, an organisation focussed on improving health through the development and implementation of health improvement programmes and the evidence base underpinning them.
4   NHS Quality Improvement Scotland, responsible for setting standards and monitoring the performance of organisations against them.
5   The Scottish Ambulance Service.
6   The State Hospitals Board, which provides care and treatment in 'conditions of special security' for patients with mental disorders.
7   The Golden Jubilee National Hospital (previously known as the National Waiting Times Centre), a private hospital purchased by NHS Scotland in

2002 to help reduce waiting times by providing a dedicated facility for elective care.

The SHED also funds support organisations, in particular National Services Scotland, which provides national and regional services to NHS Scotland organisations, such as paying family health services practitioners and providing specialist legal services, blood transfusion services, and numerous others.

Organisations planning and delivering services

UNIFIED HEALTH BOARDS

NHS Scotland is an integrated system, with a single type of organisation, unified health boards, responsible for both planning and delivering healthcare services in their areas, funded by annual budgets. They produce Local Health Plans which detail how services will be provided to improve the health of their local populations, reduce health inequalities and meet healthcare needs, while their operating divisions are responsible for providing services. The unified boards also undertake regional and Scotland-wide planning for workforce issues and specialist services through their participation in three regional planning groups.

The boards' operating divisions were formed out of Scotland's 28 self-governing trusts, which were abolished in 2004 with the abolition of the purchaser–provider split. Their former management teams were absorbed into the boards' divisional management teams. Most boards have one operating division which provides secondary (hospital) care services, and one which provides community and mental health care services and oversees the provision of family health services. Local flexibility is allowed. For example the Dumfries and Galloway health board and the Borders board each have just one operating division which provides all elements of healthcare.

Family health services are 'secured' by boards through contracts with independent practitioners – GPs, dentists, pharmacists and opticians – or provided by practitioners directly employed by the boards. The terms of service of providers of primary care are less flexible than in England, where 'personal medical services' or PMS contracts can be tailored to the circumstances of individual GPs (see Chapter 4, page 52). In Scotland all primary care services are provided under the title of 'primary medical services', with terms of provision and remuneration corresponding to the new 'general medical services' or GMS contract introduced in England in 2004.

Although foundation trusts have not been introduced in Scotland, alternatives to traditional models of secondary care provision are being introduced. These include initiatives such as the use of dedicated treatment centres to provide elective secondary care services and the national 24-hour telephone nurse triage system (NHS 24) already mentioned, to direct patients to the most appropriate form of out-of-hours care. It is also intended that services should increasingly be delivered through 'managed clinical networks'. These are linked groups of healthcare professionals and organisations to provide clear 'patient pathways' for specific conditions such as coronary heart disease and diabetes. They are intended to provide integrated services that cross organisational boundaries, as well as the geographic boundaries of health boards and regions. Ultimately they will also be extended to include elements of social care provided by local authorities, to produce 'managed care networks'.

COMMUNITY HEALTH PARTNERSHIPS

As in the English NHS, devolution of responsibility to 'frontline' organisations and staff is an important aim of NHS Scotland. The operating divisions of the unified boards are expected to delegate decision-making authority and budgetary powers to the appropriate level. In addition each board has a number of 'community health partnerships', committees or sub-committees of the board operating at local level and incorporating Scotland's former local healthcare co-operatives (voluntary groupings of general practices).

Community health partnerships consist of members of the health board, local healthcare professionals, members of the local authority and local voluntary organisations, and a member of the local public partnership forum (see below, page 163). They are intended to take part in the planning of services undertaken by health boards, and to facilitate the integration of primary/community and secondary care or hospital services through the development of managed clinical networks. They may hold delegated budgets and be responsible for managing and providing services, co-ordinating the delivery of services, and securing services from independent contractors such as GPs and dentists.

'JOINT FUTURES STRUCTURES'

One of the key roles of community health partnerships is to work with local authorities. As part of this they may be given responsibility for the 'joint futures' agenda, an initiative intended to help overcome the barriers to joint working that result from the fact that the boundaries of unified health boards and local authorities do not coincide. 'Joint futures structures', formed between either health boards or community health partnerships and the social services departments of local authorities (usually more than one), can hold pooled budgets, share assessments of patients, and jointly manage staff for the delivery of community health and social care services.

THE INDEPENDENT SECTOR

Within Scotland use of the independent (private and voluntary) sector has been introduced as a means to provide additional capacity, specifically to address waiting time targets. Although there has been explicit recognition that use of the independent sector must not detract from the duty of NHS health boards to develop

NHS services to meet the needs of the local population, the SEHD is considering making greater use of the private sector to undertake additional NHS work.

Public health

Health improvement is an important part of Scotland's health policy. There is a national directorate of health improvement within the SEHD and all the Scottish NHS boards have Directors of Public Health. The development and implementation of local health promotion services is also one of the key functions of community health partnerships.

A national body, NHS Health Scotland, has been established to encourage healthy lifestyles by acting as the national agency for health education, health promotion and health advice. It was formed as a special health board in 2003, by the amalgamation of the Health Education Board for Scotland and the Public Health Institute for Scotland. Its work involves analysing and disseminating information on health and health improvement programmes, identifying evidence to inform the development of health improvement programmes, and undertaking such programmes through advertising, publications, and the provision of training and development opportunities.

Health protection functions are overseen at national level by Health Protection Scotland, a body established in 2004. It is responsible for providing expert advice on health protection issues to government, healthcare organisations and professionals and the public. It is also responsible for monitoring health hazards or exposures and the effects they have on the population's health, and for undertaking relevant research and development activities. As well as monitoring infectious disease rates it commissions services from the 'national reference laboratories', a network of laboratories that provide specialist microbiological services. It also supports and monitors the effectiveness of the local health protection networks formed by the unified health boards and local authorities. These networks are responsible for developing joint health protection plans, such as plans to deal with outbreaks of communicable disease or 'emergency' situations such as those that could result from bio-terrorism.

Quality and regulation

Many of the mechanisms used to ensure the quality of services in the English NHS (described in Chapter 6) are also used by NHS Scotland. The exception is the commissioning process: in Scotland services are planned and delivered by a single organisation. Again unlike England, most of the mechanisms used to ensure the 'quality' of services are operated by a single independent organisation, a special health board, established in April 2003, called Quality Improvement Scotland (QIS). It has a wider remit than its English counterpart, the Healthcare Commission.

All NHS Scotland organisations are ultimately accountable to the Scottish Parliament via Scotland's Minister for Health and Community Care. The chairs of the unified health boards are answerable to the minister and their chief executives are answerable to the SEHD through its directorate of performance management and finance.

This process is linked to a system of escalating intervention for poorly-performing NHS Boards. Ministers can intervene in those deemed to be failing through a variety of mechanisms, such as a requirement to produce a recovery plan, 'strengthening' the board's management function, replacing specific staff such as the chief executive, or removing the whole board of directors. Both the chairs and the chief executives of NHS boards can also be called to account by parliamentary committees examining specific aspects of healthcare provision.

STANDARDS AND MONITORING

QIS assures standards of service delivery through a number of mechanisms. It provides advice on the clinical- and cost-effectiveness of specific treatments and medicines through health technology appraisals. It also disseminates NICE guidance (which relates to England and Wales) relating to such matters. It neither assesses nor 'approves' such guidance, but comments on it in light of the ways Scotlands' epidemiology, rurality, or structure of services differ from England's.

QIS also funds and oversees the work of the Scottish Inter-Collegiate Guidelines Network (SIGN), a multi-disciplinary working group drawn from across the medical professions. SIGN produces evidence-based national clinical guidelines for the clinical management of specific conditions, particularly those where there are known to be variations in practice within Scotland. By April 2005 it had produced, or was in the process of developing, 79 sets of guidelines.[4] The programme of National Service Frameworks (NSFs) discussed in Chapter 6 also applies to Scotland, providing frameworks or service models for the delivery of care for specific conditions or patient groups.

As in England the quality of primary care services is addressed within the 'quality and outcomes framework' of Scotland's general medical services contract, and linked to the financial remuneration of GP practices. QIS also sets standards against which to monitor the performance of other services provided by NHS boards. These cover 'generic' issues such as levels of hospital cleanliness as well as clinical indicators relating to the outcomes of particular conditions or treatments. QIS assesses performance against these standards annually, through a system of self-assessment checked or 'validated' by an inspection process involving peer review. Findings are published, so that boards can use them to improve service performance and quality.

As in England, Scotland's NHS organisations (i.e. the health boards) are required to ensure that internal mechanisms are in place to monitor and improve the quality of healthcare, i.e. to have clinical governance arrangements. The boards are supported in this by the QIS, which provides 'toolkits' and advice on best practice, as well as reviewing their arrangements and making recommendations on how to improve them.

Professional self-regulation by the professional regulatory councils – the GMC, etc. (see Chapter 6, pages 121–2) – with their systems of appraisal and ultimately revalidation, is UK-wide and so includes Scotland. Scotland, however, also has a special health board called NHS Education Scotland which provides education and training courses and other development opportunities for NHS Scotland staff. As in England, the introduction of the pay restructuring system 'Agenda for Change' has also resulted in the introduction of annual development reviews to identify the learning needs of non-medical staff.

To ensure that NHS Scotland learns from 'adverse events' these are monitored by QIS (the function performed in England by the National Patient Safety Agency, see Chapter 6, page 126). QIS is also responsible for investigating and recommending remedial action for 'serious service failures' which may come to light through the monitoring of standards or from reports by professionals or patients. However its remit does not extend to suggesting remedial action for individual professionals who are found to be performing poorly. Scotland lacks a specific agency to deal with this issue, and some chief executives of NHS boards have approached England's National Clinical Assessment Service for advice.

Patient and public involvement

As in the English NHS, the involvement of patients and the public is considered an important part of the accountability of Scotland's health services. NHS boards are required to have 'lay' non-executive members on their boards of directors. They also have a statutory duty to ensure the involvement of patients and the public in the planning and delivery of services, for example by monitoring the views of service users and by involving patients and their carers in the development of the managed care networks discussed above (page 160).

The duty to involve patients and the public also extends to community health partnerships. They are required to engage with their local communities through local 'public partnership forums', and to have at least one member of these forums on their committee. 'Public partnership forums' are 'networks' or 'virtual groupings' of existing voluntary organisations, user and carer groups, and 'interested individuals'. They are intended to provide a mechanism for the two-way flow of information between community health partnerships and patients and the public – to inform local people about local services and to gather their views and opinions on how to improve them, and to ensure that the views of local people are represented in planning and decision-making.

A body known as the Scottish Health Council, established as part of QIS, is responsible for overseeing the arrangements for involving patients and the public in health issues. As well as supporting community health partnerships and public partnership forums by providing advice, training, and development, the Council has an external scrutiny role. It monitors the arrangements of community health partnerships and can ask the relevant NHS board to take action to see that appropriate arrangements exist. It also monitors the arrangements for public participation in NHS boards, reporting to the public as well as the boards on the progress that is being made in achieving patient and public involvement. The council works through local offices in each NHS board area. Each office has an 'advisory council' made up of local volunteers who are directly involved in the scrutiny of arrangements.

The NHS in Wales

The NHS in Wales (known as NHS Wales) serves a population of almost 3 million people.[4] Its 85,000 staff include 4,600 doctors and almost 40,000 nurses, midwives and health visitors.[5] There are also some 1,900 GPs, 1,000 dentists, and 600 opticians.[6]

NHS Wales is overseen by the Wales Assembly Government, established in 1999. Unlike the devolved administrations of Scotland and Northern Ireland, the Welsh Assembly does not have the power to make primary legislation. Some Acts of the Westminster Parliament are 'Wales only' Acts and some encompass both England and Wales. The Assembly has executive powers, however, and can make secondary legislation determining policy and implementing legislation made at Westminster.

Within these constraints the Assembly produced its own version of the English NHS Plan in 2001, *Improving Health in Wales. A plan for the NHS with its Partners*. As in England, this declared the intention of moving away from the internal market of the 1990s, but retaining a 'purchaser–provider split'. Structural reforms were subsequently implemented in April 2003, under the provisions of the NHS Reform and Health Care Professions Act 2002 and the Health (Wales) Act 2003.

The structure of NHS Wales

The structure of NHS Wales is shown in Figure 9.2. Local health boards, analogous to the English PCTs, are responsible for commissioning or 'purchasing' services from provider trusts, and for overseeing the provision of family health services from GPs, dentists, etc.

Organisations with strategic roles

THE WALES ASSEMBLY GOVERNMENT AND THE NHS WALES DEPARTMENT

The Welsh Executive's Minister for Health and Social Services and the NHS Wales Department (NHSWD) are responsible for determining health policy, allocating healthcare resources and overseeing the delivery of services through NHS Wales.

The NHSWD is led by the Director of NHS Wales and undertakes its work through seven national directorates. These are responsible for:

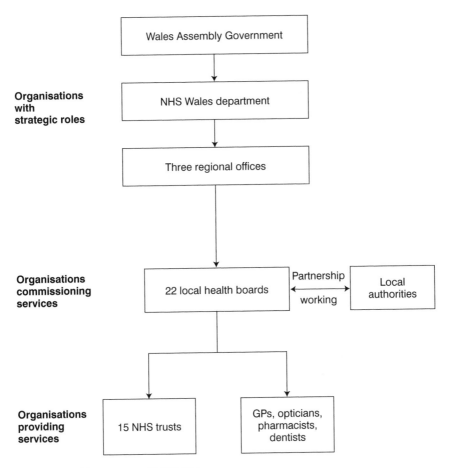

Figure 9.2   The structure of NHS Wales

1 Developing policy relating to clinical health services.
2 Overseeing the development and implementation of policies relating to primary care services.
3 Developing and implementing systems relating to the quality and regulation of services and the performance management of NHS Wales organisations.
4 Allocating financial and other resources and dealing with other financial issues such as counter-fraud policy.
5 Managing human resources issues within the department and across NHS Wales.
6 Providing health information and facilities, developing and managing the capital estate and developing information management and technology.
7 Giving 'central support' to the Welsh Assembly, such as managing responses to briefing requests and the media.

As in the DH in England, the NHSWD gets professional advice from the Chief Medical Officer and the Chief Nursing Officer. It has three regional offices (north, south and west, mid and east). Led by regional directors, these offices are responsible for ensuring that policies are implemented across their regions. They also play a strategic leadership role, for example by helping to develop networks and programmes that span more than one individual organisation. In addition, like England's SHAs (see Chapter 2, pages 18–20), they are responsible for 'performance managing' NHS organisations within their areas.

At national level the work of the NHS Wales Department is supported by the National Health and Well Being Council. The Council's role is to monitor progress in the implementation of the Welsh health plan, *Improving Health in Wales*. It also provides advice, given either by its own members or commissioned from other forums and groups, on any further action or policy development that may be needed. The Council is chaired by the Minister for Health and Social Services, and composed of NHS staff and representatives of professional bodies as well as staff drawn from social care services, local government, patient groups and the voluntary sector.

The NHSWD also has a number of 'arm's length bodies', national organisations which it funds to undertake particular functions on its behalf. Discussed in more detail below, these are the Health Commission Wales (commissioning specialist and tertiary services), the Health Inspectorate Wales (responsible for inspecting NHS organisations), the National Public Health Service (providing reference microbiological services), and the Wales Centre for Health (supporting the public health function).

Organisations commissioning services

As in England a single local organisation is responsible for securing the whole range of healthcare services for its resident population. Analogous to PCTs (see Chapter 4 pages 36–43), these are known as Local Health Boards (LHBs).

LOCAL HEALTH BOARDS

Twenty-two LHBs are responsible for improving the health of their local communities. With similar boundaries to those of local authorities they receive direct financial allocations with which to secure the whole range of health services for their local populations. This involves commissioning primary and community healthcare services, and having responsibility for developing these services. It is intended that they should become increasingly involved in directly providing these services themselves. LHBs also commission or 'purchase' hospital or secondary care services (specialist and tertiary services are commissioned nationally by the Health Commission Wales, mentioned above).

'Partnership working' is intended to be a key feature of LHBs. This is reflected in the composition of their boards, which may consist of up to 26 members, and includes representation from primary care, community care, public health, local government and local voluntary organisations, as well as 'lay' members. LHBs are required to work with local authorities to produce health, social care and well-being strategies which should involve a 'whole systems' approach to strategic and operational planning that includes the socio-economic determinants of health. Commissioning of hospital services is also to be undertaken in partnership with other organisations, namely trusts, LHBs, and local authorities, facilitated by the NHSWD's regional offices. This is intended to make it possible to develop more integrated services that cross organisational boundaries, such as 'integrated care pathways'.

Organisations providing services

Hospital and community health services are provided by 14 NHS trusts (one of which provides the all-Wales ambulance service), on the same basis as in England. Between them they manage 135 hospitals and 15,000 inpatient beds.[6] As well as providing hospital and community health services commissioned by the LHBs and the Health Commission Wales, they are also required to participate in partnership working with these and other organisations. This is intended to be a key element of commissioning arrangements, and to ensure that NHS trusts are actively involved in the development of LHBs, health, social care, and well-being strategies.

Primary care services and the other elements of family health services (dental, pharmaceutical and ophthalmic) are provided by independent practitioners, who provide services under contract to their LHB, again as in England. There are almost 1,900 GPs in Wales, as well as almost 1,000 dentists, and 600 opticians, supported by health visitors, midwives and community nurses and other staff.[6]

Integrated organisations

One LHB (Powys) was established as an integrated organisation combining both commissioner and provider functions, being an LHB that also provided community health services. Following this example there is now a programme in place to integrate a number of LHBs that commission services with trusts that provide services.

Public health

The office of the CMO reports directly to the Wales Assembly Government, providing health professional support to policy divisions within it. It also oversees the new National Public Health Service. This service has no statutory responsibility to undertake public health duties, but provides public health support to the LHBs, which are largely responsible for public health functions at the local level. This support is provided by public health laboratory and related services and dedicated public health specialists who function as corporate members of the LHBs. The office of the CMO also oversees the work of a new Wales Centre for Health. Established as an independent NHS body, its role is to support public health throughout Wales by providing training to support multi-professional development, developing the public health evidence base through research, providing health information through public health observatories, and co-ordinating the development of public health networks.

Quality and regulation

Many of the mechanisms used to ensure the quality of services in the English NHS (see Chapter 6) are also used by NHS Wales, and the remits of several organisations such as NICE and the Healthcare Commission extend to NHS Wales. In Wales, however, there is more emphasis on using the quality and regulation process to help organisations to improve their performance, rather than merely assessing their performance and expecting them to improve it themselves, as in England.

ACCOUNTABILITY ARRANGEMENTS

Accountability arrangements closely parallel those in England. All NHS Wales statutory organisations are directly accountable to the Minister for Health and Social Services and the Wales Assembly Government. Their chief executives are accountable to the Director of NHS Wales, whose regional directors 'performance manage' LHBs and NHS trusts. As in England, too, the commissioning process is intended to play a role in accountability. NHS trusts are held to account by LHBs through their long-term agreements with LHBs, and for secondary and tertiary services with Health Commission Wales.

STANDARDS AND MONITORING

National standards of service delivery are also set by the same national service frameworks (NSFs) as in England, and as already mentioned the remit of NICE (see Chapter 6, pages 113–14) extends to NHS Wales. So too does the remit of the Healthcare Commission, though only in making an assessment or 'overview' of the provision of Welsh healthcare services in its annual report to Parliament. Local review and inspection of NHS bodies is undertaken by a new NHS Wales Healthcare Inspection Unit. This is analogous to the Healthcare Commission, although it assesses the performance of NHS Wales organisations against a framework for continuous improvement rather than against a set of performance standards. The continuous improvement framework does not try to encapsulate performance within a few indicators, and also considers local pressures and the availability of local resources. By identifying areas for improvement it attempts to 'steer' organisations in improving and sustaining performance.

As in England, the quality of primary care services is specifically addressed within the quality and outcomes framework of the general medical services contract, and linked to financial remuneration for GP practices. There are also several mechanisms for ensuring the provision of quality services at local level.

As in England, all NHS organisations are required to ensure that mechanisms are in place to monitor and improve the quality of healthcare – again as in England – through clinical governance arrangements. The professional self-regulation system operating in England also applies to Wales, as do the Agenda for Change (see Chapter 6) and annual development reviews to identify learning needs for non-medical staff.

NHS Wales falls within the remit of the National Patient Safety Agency. As discussed in Chapter 6, this organisation provides a reporting and feedback system to ensure that NHS organisations and the NHS learn from adverse incidents. As part of this NHS organisations in Wales can use the services of the National Clinical Assessment Service (see Chapter 6, pages 122–3), providing advice, support, and remedial action such as re-training for healthcare professionals found to be poorly performing.

Patient and public involvement

As in the English NHS the involvement of patients and the public is considered an important element in the accountability of services. Thus LHBs and NHS trusts are required to ensure that the views of local voluntary organisations and local residents are considered as part of working in partnerships to develop health, social care, and well-being strategies. Public representation is achieved through representation of local voluntary groups and local or 'lay' people on their boards of directors, but also through the work of Community Health Councils (CHCs). In England CHCs were abolished by the NHS Reform and Healthcare Professions Act 2002, but in Wales they were re-established by the NHS (Wales) Act 2003. There are 20 CHCs in Wales, based roughly on local authority areas, consisting of volunteers drawn from the local community to represent patients and the public, with budgets to cover some support staff and other resources. They take up a wide range of health issues, and LHBs are required to consult them over proposed major changes in services. Their work also incorporates a patient support and advocacy role in relation to complaints.

The NHS in Northern Ireland

The NHS in Northern Ireland serves a population of approximately 1.7 million.[7] It has some 54,000 staff, the largest group being its 15,000 midwives and nursing staff, with just over 3,200 medical and dental staff, as well as 4,500 staff providing social care services (as explained below, in Northern Ireland the provision of social services is integrated with the provision of health services).[8]

Since political devolution in 1999 the NHS in Northern Ireland has fallen under the jurisdiction of the Northern Ireland Assembly, which like Scotland's Parliament can pass primary legislation on devolved matters and can amend or repeal Acts of the UK Parliament in so far as they touch on matters within the Assembly's jurisdiction. The Assembly's Executive is responsible for determining health policy, for allocating healthcare resources, and overseeing the delivery of healthcare services.

The suspension of devolution in October 2002, however, meant that responsibility for the Northern Ireland departments (including health and social care) passed for the time being back to the Northern Ireland Office in London, headed by the Secretary of State for Northern Ireland and a team of junior ministers.

Against this background policy development and organisational reform of the NHS in Northern Ireland has been limited. In 2000 a Northern Ireland equivalent of the NHS Plan, *Investing in Health*, was published, which laid emphasis on the need for partnerships between health, social care, and other organisations. The 2001 Health and Personal Social Services Act (Northern Ireland) subsequently provided for the establishment of local health and social care groups to provide a 'local dimension' in the planning and commissioning of services.

Proposals for further re-organisation were laid out in a consultation document in June 2002, entitled *Developing Better Services: Modernising Hospitals and Reforming Structures*. Options proposed included the devolution of commissioning to consortia of local health and social care groups (akin to PCTs in England, but with responsibility for social care as well as health care), and the amalgamation of commissioners and providers within an integrated body (as in Scotland). But since the suspension of devolution these proposals have remained under consideration; re-organisation is currently limited to the re-organisation of hospital services in order to provide a network of hospitals specialising in acute and elective care.

The structure of the NHS in Northern Ireland

The NHS in Northern Ireland is unique within the UK in that since the 1970s it has provided both health and social care services. This is the task of 'Health and Personal Social Services' or HPSS, an organisation overseen by the Department of Health, Social Services and Public Safety (DHSSPS). Despite this its structure is broadly similar to that of the NHS in England, organised around a 'purchaser–provider split' (see Figure 9.3).

Organisations with strategic roles

THE NORTHERN IRELAND EXECUTIVE AND THE DEPARTMENT OF HEALTH, SOCIAL SERVICES AND PUBLIC SAFETY

Since devolution was suspended the minister for health and personal social services in the Northern Ireland Office has been responsible for overseeing the HPSS, in place of the Northern Ireland Executive. The HPSS is the Northern Ireland equivalent of the NHS and covers primary, secondary and community care. It is overseen by the DHSSPS, which as its name suggests, also covers issues such as public safety (e.g. emergency planning) and health promotion (which is also true of the analogous bodies in England and the other devolved countries,

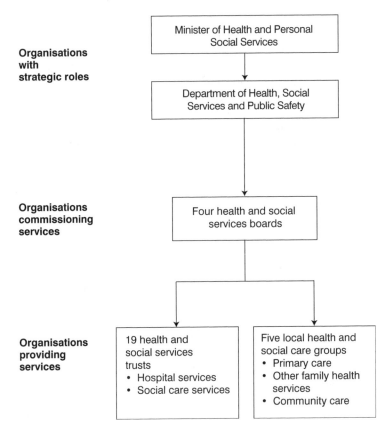

Organisations with strategic roles

Minister of Health and Personal Social Services

↓

Department of Health, Social Services and Public Safety

Organisations commissioning services

Four health and social services boards

Organisations providing services

19 health and social services trusts
- Hospital services
- Social care services

Five local health and social care groups
- Primary care
- Other family health services
- Community care

Figure 9.3   The structure of health and personal social services (the NHS) in Northern Ireland.

although not similarly reflected in their titles); but it is the department responsible for overseeing the provision of health services, through the HPSS. Each year the DHSSPS issues 'priorities for action' by the HPSS, laying out priority areas and targets.

The DHSSPS is organised into three work areas or 'groups'. These are:

1   The planning and resources group, responsible for preparing the overall strategic plan for health services, for managing financial and staff resources, and for issues relating to public safety such as planning for ambulance services and emergency situations.
2   The hospital and personal social services management group, responsible for developing 'operational policy' to 'modernise' services, and for monitoring and managing the performance of services.
3   The primary, secondary and community care group, responsible for developing and overseeing the implementation of policies relating to the commissioning and delivery of these services.

There are also five professional groups, each led by a chief professional officer, providing advice and specific functions such as the inspection of services or the provision of prison dental services; medical and allied services (e.g. physiotherapy and radiography); the social services inspectorate; nursing and midwifery services; dental services; and pharmaceutical services.

The DHSSPS also has an executive agency called Health Estates, funded by and accountable to it but functioning autonomously. It provides advice and support on all matters relating to the land, buildings and equipment of the NHS in Northern Ireland, advising ministers and NHS organisations on issues such as fire safety, capital development plans and specific projects, and setting standards for, and issuing guidance on, new buildings. It also provides services such as inspecting sites to ensure that standards are met, and handling the transaction process when estate is sold, purchased or leased.

As in England and the other devolved countries there are a number of other agencies, also funded by the DHSSPS but independent from it, which provide specific functions on its behalf. These are:

- The HPSS Regulation and Improvement Authority (RIA), which inspects and reports on the quality of services delivered by the HPSS against standards set by the department.
- The Central Services Agency, which provides specialist services such as financial services (central banking arrangements and the payment of independent family health services practitioners on behalf of NHS organisations), and legal services relating to areas such as employment law and medical negligence claims.
- The Health Promotion Agency, which provides leadership, support, and information for those working in health promotion.
- The Blood Transfusion Agency, which is responsible for collecting, testing, and distributing blood and blood products.
- The Regional Medical Physics Agency, supporting trusts by providing health and social care services in matters relating to the use of radiation and radioactive material.
- The Guardian Ad Litem Agency, which provides independent social work investigation and support and represents the interests of children during legal proceedings relating to care or supervision orders, emergency protection orders, and the placement of young people in secure accommodation.

Organisations commissioning services

HEALTH AND SOCIAL SERVICES BOARDS

In Northern Ireland both health and personal social services are organised around a 'purchaser–provider split'. The four regional health and social services boards (east, north, west and south) are responsible for assessing both the health and the social care needs of their resident populations. They are also responsible for 'purchasing' services to meet those needs, by commissioning hospital and community health and social care services from trusts, and overseeing the provision of family health services through contracts with GPs, dentists and other providers – or by directly employing family health service practitioners to provide them.

Since April 2002, 15 Local Health and Social Care Groups (LHSCGs) have been responsible for planning and delivering primary and social care services in their areas. Replacing GP fundholders, they operate as 'committees' of the local health and social services board, and are based on groups of GP practices, serving populations ranging from 60,000 to 200,000.[9] Their members include representatives of the local health and social care board, trusts providing local hospital and community services, and GPs, nurses, social workers, pharmacists and allied health professionals, as well as local community and service users.

LHSCGs are responsible for planning and delivering both health and social care services outside the hospital setting, including those delivered by health visitors, district nurses, allied health professionals and social workers, as well as those provided by GPs, dentists, community pharmacists and optometrists. They are intended to facilitate partnership working between health and social care organisations, and to provide a mechanism for community involvement in the planning and delivery of services.

Their remit also includes contributing to their local health and social care board and helping to make commissioning decisions for hospital and community health and social care services, and as they develop they are assuming greater responsibility in this area. Becoming more like English primary care trusts, a number of them are now responsible for commissioning specific hospital and/or community services, receiving budgets for this purpose from their health boards.

Organisations providing services

HOSPITAL AND COMMUNITY HEALTH AND SOCIAL SERVICES

Hospital and community health and social care services are provided by 19 trusts, whose services are commissioned or 'purchased' by health and social services boards (and increasingly by LHSCGS). Some of the 19 trusts provide hospital services only, some provide community health and social services only, and some provide both, while one provides ambulance services across Northern Ireland. Following the 2002 consultation document, *Developing Better Services: Modernising Hospitals and Reforming Structures*, hospital services are being re-organised to provide a network of nine acute hospitals so that most of the population will be within 45 minutes of emergency care and consultant-led maternity services, supplemented by a number of 'enhanced local hospitals' and a specialist centre providing stand-alone elective surgery.

PRIMARY CARE SERVICES

Primary care services are provided through some 350 GP practices, along with their associated health visitors, district nurses and allied health professionals. They are generally provided under contract to health and social services boards, although these boards are now able to employ practitioners directly. The other elements of family health services – dental, community pharmacy, and ophthalmic services – are, as in England, provided by independent practitioners working under contract with the health boards.

THE INDEPENDENT SECTOR

The independent (private and voluntary) sector has traditionally provided a relatively small proportion of health care services (as opposed to social care services where they are important providers of nursing and residential care-home services). The DHSSPS has stated that it has 'no immediate plans' to follow the English example of using the independent sector as a major provider of elective surgical procedures, but will 'closely monitor developments and seek to learn from the experience'.[10]

Public health

The public health work of the DHSSPS is supported by two agencies, the Health Promotion Agency and the Communicable Disease Surveillance Centre. The Health Promotion Agency focuses on areas of work such as nutrition, physical activity, smoking cessation, and sexual health. It provides advice to the DHSSPS and other government departments and undertakes research to evaluate the effectiveness of health promotion policies and interventions. It also provides training activities for health promotion staff, produces health promotion publications, and undertakes health promotion campaigns.

The Communicable Disease Surveillance Centre (Northern Ireland) is a branch of the English Health Protection Agency (see Chapter 2, page 33). It monitors communicable diseases and provides support and advice to staff in health and social services boards in dealing with communicable diseases, outbreaks, and major incidents.

All four health and social services boards have Directors of Public Health. They are responsible for taking the lead on health promotion issues and for ensuring that emergency planning is undertaken and that systems are in place for the prevention, surveillance and control of communicable diseases. The last of these tasks is usually delegated to a locally-employed consultant in communicable disease control.

Quality and regulation

Following a 2001 consultation document entitled *Best Care, Best Practice*, mechanisms similar to those used in the English NHS (see Chapter 6) have been adopted in Northern Ireland, although many of them are at an earlier stage of development than their English counterparts.

ACCOUNTABILITY ARRANGEMENTS

So long as devolution remains suspended all Northern Ireland's NHS organisations are ultimately accountable to the Westminster Parliament, although accountability still runs through the DHSSPS in Belfast. The DHSSPS holds Health and Social Services Boards and the trusts directly to account (i.e. there are no SHAs, as in England) for the effective and efficient use of their resources and for their arrangements to engage users, carers and the wider community. Local Health and Social Care Groups are committees of Health and Social Care Boards, and as such are directly accountable to them.

As in England the commissioning process also plays a role in accountability. Health and Social Care Boards are responsible for ensuring the quality and performance of the services they commission.

STANDARDS AND MONITORING

There are a number of mechanisms through which standards of service delivery are set and maintained for the HPSS in Northern Ireland. Guidelines produced by the National Institute for Health and Clinical Excellence (NICE), which relate to the clinical and cost-effectiveness of treatments and medicines, are only applicable to England and Wales, but as in Scotland they are recognised as a resource by the DHSSPS, which advises health and social services boards and trusts on their local applicability. An advisory committee of healthcare professionals (doctors, nurses, and allied health professionals) analogous to SIGN in Scotland, called the Clinical Resource Efficiency Support Team or CREST, also produces guidelines on the management of specific clinical conditions, such as chronic heart failure or resistant depression.

The DHSSPS is in the process of developing a set of standards for providers of health and social care which will eventually encompass all aspects of service delivery, organisation, and management. New standards developed by the DHSSPS are monitored by the HPSS's Regulation and Improvement Authority (RIA), mentioned earlier. Becoming fully operational in 2005 the RIA, although funded by the DHSSPS, is a non-departmental public body charged with inspecting and reporting on the services provided by both HPSS organisations (trusts) and independent sector providers (in Northern Ireland, predominantly providers of social care services).

As in England and the other devolved countries the remit of the RIA does not extend to independent practitioners providing family health services. The quality of primary care services is addressed within the 'quality and outcomes framework' of the general medical services contract or GMS, and linked to the financial remuneration of GP practices.

Again as in England, all HPSS organisations are under a statutory duty of quality. They are required to put in place clinical governance arrangements to monitor and improve the quality of services. The DHSSPS assists them through an NHS clinical governance support team, which provides services such as training for staff.

As already noted, the UK's professional regulatory councils and their requirements for appraisal and revalidation cover the whole of the UK and so include Northern Ireland, as does the NHS pay restructuring system 'Agenda for Change' which has led to the introduction of annual development reviews to identify learning needs for non-medical staff.

As in the other devolved countries, learning from adverse events has been recognised as an important part of the quality agenda. A voluntary system for reporting incidents relating to medical devices is run by the Northern Ireland Adverse Incident Centre. The HPSS lacks a system for reporting incidents relating to other kinds adverse medical incident, such as errors by medical staff, but is in the process of developing links with the English National Patient Safety Agency, described in Chapter 6 (see page 126). The HPSS also lacks any equivalent to the English National Clinical Assessment Service, which suggests remedial action for individual professionals found to be performing poorly.

Patient and public involvement

The boards of directors of health and social care boards and trusts, and the committees of local health and social services groups, contain non-executive directors drawn from the local community, to represent the views and concerns of patients and the public. The involvement of patients and the public is also addressed through independent Health and Social Service Councils. These Councils, one for each of the four health and social services board areas, are independent 'consumer' organisations funded by the DHSSPS. Their role is to represent the views of service users on issues relating to the planning and delivery of services, to review the work of health and social service organisations in their areas, and to recommend any improvements needed.

Summary

England, Wales and Northern Ireland all employ the so-called 'purchaser–provider split', whereby local organisations commission or 'purchase' hospital and community services on behalf of their resident populations. The commissioning organisations also oversee the provision of family health services through contracts with independent practitioners, although they can now provide such services themselves using directly employed staff.

England stands alone, however, in having introduced a new financial framework ('payment by results') that seeks to reward providers of care for the volume of work actually undertaken, increasingly determined by the choices patients make about where to go for elective treatment. England also stands alone in introducing the independent sector as a mainstream provider of NHS services. Wales and Northern Ireland, while retaining the English model of 'the purchaser–provider split', have not adopted the policy of 'foundation' status for providers, or 'payments by results'.

Scotland stands alone in having abandoned the 'purchase–provider split' and having abolished the semi-autonomous trusts which contract to 'sell' hospital and community health services to 'purchasers'. Its policy of re-integrating the trusts with the bodies that previously commissioned services contrasts most sharply with policy in England, where trusts providing services are being granted still greater autonomy and freedoms, above all through foundation status.

Northern Ireland stands alone in integrating health and social care services under a single central ministry.

Over time these differences seem likely to give rise to others. A case in point is differences in the terms of service for doctors in each country. Mention has already been made of the fact that PMS contracts for GPs in England are not available to GPs in Scotland. The formula for distributing GP practices' 'global sums' also varies from country to country. In the new consultants' contract, too, the standard working week, the basic salary scale and salary progression in England are different from those in Wales, while Scotland has retained the old system of 'discretionary points' and distinction awards which have been replaced in England by Clinical Excellence Awards. Unless steps are taken to ensure that such differences do not come to pose significant barriers, some decline in professional contacts and movements of staff between the countries of the UK seems likely to occur.

10 The future

The new NHS is still taking shape, with further changes to its structures and functions announced as this book was being finalised. Plans are well advanced for mergers and reconfigurations of PCTs and SHAs. Crucially, the DH White Paper *Our Health, Our Care*, published in January 2006, made it clear that the government intends to contract out to the private sector the commissioning functions and budgets of PCTs through 'practice-based' commissioning.[1] Under practice-based commissioning providers of GP services will hold the budgets and commission all medical services, including primary care, community health services and hospital care. The DH is working with a number of large corporations, and PCTs are contracting with US companies like UnitedHealth Europe and Kaiser Permanente to operate GP practices and provide community health services;[2] through practice-based commissioning they will become the health care commissioners for the patients in their care.

Meanwhile Mid Surrey PCT has seen the first management buyout of community health services by NHS staff.[3] Acute services are also being privatized, with the planned transfer to private providers of 15 per cent of all NHS elective surgery, and the further planned transfer of other services, including radiology and pathology. This process will accelerate with the introduction of practice-based commissioning, which will give private providers control over a significant proportion of PCT budgets, which currently account for 80 per cent of all NHS funds. The day when the NHS becomes mainly a mere funder of health care – a 'logo' attached to the provision of health care by private hospitals and surgeries – no longer seems remote.

With so much at stake, it is important not only to try to understand what is happening, but also to ask questions about it. The central issues clearly concern two things. First how far the new NHS will, or can, continue to serve the values and aims of the original NHS, namely services which are universal, comprehensive and free at the point of delivery. Second, how far the market-based system, adopted for the sake of efficiency, will actually be more efficient than what it is replacing.

As regards the core NHS value of universality, for example, we might ask what mechanisms will ensure that the progressive equalization of resources and services, on the basis of population need, throughout the different parts of the UK, will be maintained. The aim is that PCTs will reach their 'target' financial allocations by

2010. But the old mechanisms for ensuring greater equity of resource allocation and service distribution no longer exist. They took into account past measures of service supply as well as indicators of patient and population need when distributing funds. Under the new system, control over resource allocation will be devolved to private or voluntary sector commissioners with no responsibility to meet the healthcare needs of a defined population.

These commissioners may both purchase and provide services to the patients on GP practice lists. Whether they are for-profit or non-profit organisations, the logic of the incentive system is that providers will try to concentrate on the most profitable treatments, services and patients, and avoid the least profitable; while commissioners will attempt to constrain costs by restricting access to care, or by capping the price (as the national tariff does now).

Some commissioners and some providers will be liable to make losses, and have to cut services and reduce entitlements to health care, because they happen to have inherited more expensive plant, or have a more expensive case-mix, or for other reasons. As this book neared publication many NHS trusts were reporting serious financial deficits, causing them to suspend or delay treatment or even close services.[4] Across the country community hospitals are closing, and major cuts are occurring in mental health services and palliative care. These cuts are making existing inequalities worse, both across areas, and between and within patient groups.

A related issue is whether any part of the NHS is now responsible for relating services to needs and ensuring universal access. In the past, public health departments within health authorities and then PCTs were responsible for gathering and analysing the healthcare needs presented by the social and economic conditions of their local populations, and for planning, monitoring and providing the requisite services accordingly. If budgets are contracted out to for-profit providers, where will the incentive to do this come from? As the pressures of market competition make themselves felt providers will close unprofitable services in order to avoid financial deficits. It is unclear how patients in the area served by those services will continue to have the same access to that service as patients elsewhere.

Second, as regards comprehensiveness, what mechanism will ensure that services for patients with conditions that are inherently hard to predict and relatively costly to treat – older patients with several chronic diseases, or the frail elderly, for example – will continue to be provided? The NHS no longer provides truly comprehensive care. Much social care and long-term care formerly provided by the NHS is now means tested and charged for, involving serious inequities in provision. Now patients' entitlements to NHS care are also being curtailed, though in a piecemeal manner, as PCTs and hospital trusts respond to market pressures, making services less available to their local populations.[5] The highly-publicized removal from the waiting list of an Oxford hospital of patients waiting for cardiac ablation, the procedure undergone by Tony Blair in 2004 to correct his irregular heart beat, is but one example.[6] Less well-documented are the effects brought about by the closure of service for mental health, palliative care, pain relief and therapies such as speech and occupational therapy services. There is no system of artificial incentives that would ensure these services remain profitable enough to meet the commercial imperatives of the shareholders and competing stakeholder interests on the boards of trusts.

Third, as regards the provision of services free at the point of delivery: if many trusts and foundation trusts continue to find themselves in persistent deficits, what will stop this leading to a new demand (from all quarters) to find additional sources of funding in the form of 'user fees' – for so-called 'hotel costs' in hospitals, or for 'enhanced services'? As is already the case for NHS dental services, routine ophthalmic services, and long-term care, a 'half way house' is beginning to emerge where NHS patients are invited to supplement their NHS care by paying a 'top-up' fee. Recent examples include maternity care, where patients can opt to buy a 'superior' package of care, covering services which were once free to all women in labour, and MRI scans and dermatology, where patients bypass the waiting-list by paying for them privately.[7]

Advocates of the market frequently advocate compulsory user fees or 'co-payments', or 'top-up insurance', whereby those who can afford it take out insurance to cover the fees, while those who cannot make do with whatever 'basic' services remain free (or do without, as many already do for dentistry and eye care and long-term care). Another proposal is vouchers, whereby every patient would receive an equal entitlement to a fixed amount of treatment, but have to pay for additional care. Vouchers are already government policy for the young disabled, and the 2006 White Paper proposes to extend their use in social care and long-term care, so it is not hard to envisage their use being extended to NHS care more generally.

Once the market is in full operation, then, 'topping-up' of one kind or another is likely to follow, undermining all the goals of the NHS. Many of the major healthcare corporations bidding to become 'mainstream' providers of NHS care are from the US where user fees, and health plans that allow users to choose the level of service they can afford to pay, are the rule. 'Choice', which is a key feature of the new NHS, is set to move from choice of service provider to choice of level of service, depending on what the individual patient is willing – and able – to pay.

As regards efficiency, it will no doubt never be possible to draw up a convincing balance sheet comparing the old and the new NHS, but since the main reason given for the change is to increase efficiency, questions about it are obviously central.

For example, first, are the incentives to save money and find more efficient ways of working, which the market is intended to encourage, compatible with good health care? Given that much of the healthcare budget is spent on staff and so much healthcare is labour-intensive, depending on thousands of interactions between patients and highly-trained and experienced clinicians, how far can 'business efficiency' be expected to improve the balance sheets without downgrading the service provided through reductions in funding of levels and quality of staff? The outsourcing of ancillary services, like hospital cleaning and catering, has yet to provide evidence that the profit motive leads to better service, or lower costs.

Second, do the gains from adopting a 'business-like' approach to service provision outweigh the costs involved in operating in a market such as making and monitoring contracts, paying for capital, invoicing and accounting for every completed treatment, marketing services, and dealing with fraud (which invariably increases with more and more complex chains of market exchanges, and is rife in US healthcare).[8] The high costs of the PFI, often defended as a way of securing 'private-sector efficiencies' for the NHS, have finally caused the government to question its efficacy in the face of spiralling costs and affordability problems, and to order a fundamental review of the PFI hospital programme.[9] In the US healthcare market, administrative costs are generally estimated to be around 20 per cent of total healthcare spending – more than three times the share consumed by administration in the NHS before the drive to marketize it.[10]

Third, how will the answers to any questions about efficiency be known if the financial operations of foundation trusts, as well as of the private sector providers and commissioners which are to become part of the NHS 'mainstream', are treated as 'commercially confidential' (as the independent regulator, Monitor, has already decided some of them will be). When all NHS trusts have become foundation trusts, and a large proportion of NHS funds are in the hands of for-profit commissioners, who will ensure that the billions of pounds of public money spent on them are publicly accounted for – apart from the independent regulator, who reports to the Secretary of State for Health, but is not answerable to him?

All these questions raise the central question of public accountability. The January 2006 White Paper includes proposals to further limit the duty laid on public bodies to consult over proposed service changes and closures, including decisions to contract out commissioning, budgets and associated clinical services to for-profit corporations. Even legal challenge, the last resort available to the public over the decisions public authorities make, is to be removed. Will any avenue then remain for the public to challenge the decisions made by private bodies and shareholders on their behalf?

This book does not offer answers to any of these questions, but anyone interested in the new NHS is bound to ask questions of this kind. We hope that the short list sketched here may provide a useful starting-point for doing so.

Notes

1 Introduction

1 *New Life for Health: The Commission on the NHS*, chaired by Will Hutton, London: Vintage, 2000, p. 1.
2 Department of Health, *Annual Report 2005*, p. 55.
3 Department of Health, 'Private finance initiative', online at <http://www.dh.gov.uk/ProcurementAndProposals/PublicPrivatePartnership/PrivateFinanceInitiative/fs/en>. (Accessed 3 January 2006).

2 Organisations with strategic roles

1 Department of Health (2004) *Departmental Report 2004*, London: The Stationery Office, p. 7, online at <http://www.dh.gov.uk/assetRoot/04/08/09/44/04080944.pdf> (Accessed 8 January 2005).
2 Ibid., p. 112, Figure 8.1 and 8.2.
3 Ibid., pp. 112–13.
4 Department of Health, 'Change programme. What has changed so far', online at <http://www.dh.gov.uk/AboutUs/AboutTheDepartment/DepartmentChangeArticle/fs/en?CONTENT_ID=4055959&chk=SInxka> (Accessed 3 November 2004).
5 NHS Modernisation Board (2004), *Caring in Many Ways, The NHS Modernisation Board's Annual Report, 2004*, London: Department of Health, Appendix 1.
6 Department of Health, 'New health authority boundaries', press release 2001/0628. This official figure would appear to be a slight underestimate of the average for England as a whole. Department of Health, 'New health authority boundaries', press release 2001/0628. 18 December 2001.
7 Cheshire and Merseyside Strategic Health Authority, *Franchise Plan 2002–2005*, Cheshire, p. 6.
8 The United Kingdom Parliament, 'Minutes of evidence taken before Health Committee Public Expenditure 2004, uncorrected evidence of oral transcript, 28 October 2004, Q. 44', online at <http://www.publications.parliament.uk/pa/cm/cmhealth.htm> (Accessed 7 December 2005).
9 Department of Health (2004), *Reconfiguring the Department of Health's Arm's Length Bodies*, London: The Stationery Office, pp. 3 and 6.
10 Ibid., p. 35.
11 Department of Health (2004), *Departmental Report 2004*, Annex B and C.
12 Department of Health (2004), *An Implementation Framework for Reconfiguring the DH Arm's Length Bodies, Redistributing Resources to the NHS Frontline*, London: The Stationery Office, p. 39.
13 Department of Health, *Departmental Report 2004*, London, p. 31.

14 The NHS Litigation Authority, 'About the NHS Litigation Authority', online at <http://www.nhsla.com/home.htm> (Accessed 9 March 2005).
15 Healthcare Commission (2005), *Strategic Plan 2005/2006*, London, p. 31. See also the Commission's website: <http://www.healthcarecommission.org.uk> (Accessed 7 December 2005).
16 Department of Health, 'NHS appointments commission', online at <http://www.dh.gov.uk/PolicyAndGuidance/HumanResourcesAndTraining/Modernising ProfessionalRegulation/NHSAppointmentsCommission/fs/en?CONTENT_ID= 4052361&chk=wiAWEy> (Accessed 9 November 2004).
17 'FHSAA decisions issued July 2004–July 2005', online at <http://www.fhsaa.org.uk/fhsaa/index.html> (Accessed 26 August 2005).

3 Organisations commissioning services

1 Department of Health, personal communication, 2002.
2 Department of Health (2004), *The NHS Improvement Plan,* p. 56.
3 Department of Health (2004), *Departmental Report 2004*, p. 90.
4 Department of Health (2004), *The NHS Improvement Plan*, p. 70.
5 Department of Health (2004), *National Standards Local Action, Health and Social Care Standards and Planning Framework*, London, Department of Health, p. 9 and Annex B.
6 Department of Health (2003), *Guidance on Commissioning Arrangements for Specialised Services*, London: The Stationery Office, p. 1.
7 Department of Health (2004), *Prison Health, Transfer of Commissioning Responsibilities to PCTs, Transfer Approval Process for April 2005*, London: The Stationery Office, p. 1.
8 Department of Health (2004), *The NHS Improvement Plan*, p. 69.
9 House of Commons Health Committee (2004), *Public Expenditure on Health and Personal Social Services 2004*, London: The Stationery Office, Table 3.8.1.
10 NHS Appointments Commission (n.d.) *The Appointment of Chairs and Non-Executives of Primary Care Trusts*, Leeds: NHS Appointments Commission.
11 Department of Health (2004), *The NHS Improvement Plan*, p. 69.
12 Northumberland Care Trust website, online at <http://www.northumberlandcaretrust.nhs.uk/site.htm> (Accessed 23 November 2004).
13 Bradford District Care Trust, 'Corporate information', online at <http://www.bdct.nhs.uk> (Accessed 23 November 2004).

4 Organisations providing services

1 House of Commons Health Committee (2004), *Public Expenditure on Health and Personal Social Services 2004*, London: The Stationery Office, Table 3.1.3.
2 Department of Health (May 2004), *Chief Executive's Report to the NHS*, London: The Stationery Office, p. 4.
3 Department of Health (December 2004), *Chief Executive's Report to the NHS*, London: The Stationery Office, p. 6.
4 Department of Health (2001), *Public Private Partnerships in the NHS. Modernising Primary Care in the NHS – NHS Local Improvement Finance Trust (LIFT) Prospectus*, London: Department of Health, p. 32.
5 Department of Health (2005), *Statistics for General Medical Practitioners in England: 1994–2004*, London: Department of Health, pp. 2 and Table 1b, online, at <www.dh.gov.uk/PublicationsandStatistics/Statistics/StatisticalWorkAreas/Worforce/fs/en> (Accessed 20 April 2005).
6 Department of Health (2005), *General Practitioner Recruitment, Retention and Vacancy Survey 2004 England and Wales*, p. 3, online at <www.dh.gov.uk/Publications

andStatistics/Statistics/StatisticalWorkAreas/Worforce/fs/en> (Accessed 20 April 2005).

7 Royal College of General Practitioners (2003), *The Primary Healthcare Team*, information sheet no. 21, London: Royal College of General Practitioners.

8 Department of Health (December 2004), *Chief Executive's Report to the NHS*, p. 12, Table D.

9 Department of Health (2003), *Practitioners with Special Interests*, London: The Stationery Office, p. 4.

10 Department of Health (May 2004), *Chief Executive's Report to the NHS*, p. 5.

11 Department of Health (December 2004), *Chief Executive's Report to the NHS*, p. 12.

12 Department of Health (2004), *2005–2006 Primary Medical Services Allocation*, AWP(05–06)PCT15, Leeds, Annex B.

13 Department of Health (2004), *Sustaining Innovation Through New PMS Arrangements*, London: The Stationery Office, p. 3.

14 Department of Health (2004), *Departmental Report 2004*, p. 62.

15 Department of Health (2004), *Establishing an NHS Walk In Centre*, London: The Stationery Office, online at <http://www.dh.gov.uk/policyandguidance/patientchoice> (Accessed 8 December 2004).

16 Department of Health (December 2004), *Chief Executive's Report to the NHS*, p. 7.

17 University of Bristol (2002), *The National Evaluation of NHS Walk-in Centres. Final Report*, Bristol: Division of Primary Health Care, University of Bristol, Chapter 7.

18 Department of Health (2005), *NHS Direct Commissioning Framework April 2005– March 2006*, London: The Stationery Office, pp. 12.

19 Laing and Buisson (2004), *Laing's Healthcare Market Review, 2004–2005*, London: Laing and Buisson, p. 173.

20 Ibid., p. 170.

21 Ibid., p. 167.

22 NHS in England, online at <http://www.nhs.uk/england/dentists/howdoifind.cmsx> (Accessed 7 December 2005).

23 Department of Health (2004), *NHS Dentistry: Delivering Change, a Report by the Chief Dental Officer (England)*, London: The Stationery Office, p. 6.

24 Department of Health, 'General dental service, selected statistics', Table B1, online at <http://www.performance.doh.gov.uk/HPSSS/TBL_B1.HTM> (Accessed 7 December 2004).

25 Department of Health (2004), *Report of the Primary Care Dental Workforce Review*, London: Department of Health, p. 5.

26 J. Reid, Secretary of State for Health (January 2004), *Ministerial Statement Concerning the Timing of Implementation of the New Contract for Dentists*, London: Department of Health.

27 Department of Health (2004), *NHS Dentistry: Delivering Change, a Report by the Chief Dental Officer (England)*, p. 2.

28 Department of Health (2003), *Ophthalmic Statistics for England, 1993–94 to 2003– 04*, London: The Stationery Office, p. 1.

29 Department of Health (2004), *Departmental Report 2004*, p. 101.

30 Department of Health (2003), *Proposals to Reform and Modernise the NHS (Pharmaceuticals Services) Regulations 1992*, London: The Stationery Office, p. 33.

31 Ibid., p. 61.

32 Department of Health (December 2004), *Chief Executive's Report to the NHS*, p. 7.

33 Department of Health (2004), *Departmental Report 2004*, p. 102.

34 Department of Health (2003), *Proposals to Reform and Modernise the NHS (Pharmaceuticals Services) Regulations 1992*, p. 1.

35 Department of Health (May 2004), *Chief Executives Report to the NHS*, statistical supplement, p. 20.

36 Department of Health (2004), *Patient Care in the Community NHS District Nursing Summary Information for 2003–2004 England*, London: The Stationery Office, p. 1.
37 Department of Health (2004), *NHS Health Visiting: Professional Advice and Support in the Community – Summary Information for 2003–04 England*, London: The Stationery Office, p. 1.
38 Department of Health (2004), *The NHS Improvement Plan*, pp. 37–8.
39 Department of Health (2004), *NHS Funded Nursing Care Allocations 2004/2005*, London: The Stationery Office, p. 10.
40 House of Commons Health Committee (2004), *Public Expenditure on Health and Personal Social Services 2003*, London: House of Commons, Question 4.16.
41 Department of Health (2004), *Departmental Report 2004*, pp. 34 and 35.
42 Department of Health (2003), *Guidance on Commissioning Arrangements for Specialised Services*, London: The Stationery Office, p. 1.
43 Department of Health (2004), *'Choose & Book' – Patient's Choice of Hospital and Booked Appointment*, London: The Stationery Office, p. 3.
44 Healthcare Commission (2004), *NHS Performance Ratings 2004/2005*, London, p. 5.
45 Department of Health, 'Bed availability and occupancy, England, 2003–04', online at <http://www.performance.doh.gov.uk/hospitalactivity/data_requests/beds_open_overnight.htm> (Accessed 20 December 2004).
46 Department of Health (2005), *Departmental Report 2005*, London: The Stationery Office, Figure 7.1, online at <http://www.dh.gov.uk/assetRoot/04/11/71/54/04117154.pdf> (Accessed 3 September 2005).
47 Laing and Buisson (2004), *Laing's Healthcare Market Review, 2004–2005*, p. 83.
48 Ibid., pp. 80 and 84.
49 House of Commons Health Committee (2003), *Public Expenditure on Health and Personal Social Services 2003*, London: House of Commons, Question 1.3.4, Table 2.
50 Department of Health, 'NHS management costs after shifting the balance of power', online at <http://www.dh.gov.uk/policyandguidance/organisationpolicy/financenadplanning/nhsmanagmentcosts> (Accessed 14 December 2004).
51 House of Commons Health Committee (2004), *Public Expenditure on Health and Personal Social Services 2004*, London: House of Commons, Table 3.8.1.
52 Monitor, Independent Regulator of NHS Foundation Trusts, 'NHS foundation trusts', online at <http://www.regulator-nhsft.gov.uk/register_nhsft.php> (Accessed 7 September 2005).
53 Monitor, Independent Regulator of NHS Foundation Trusts, 'NHS foundation trusts: Next applicants', online at <http://www.regulator-nhsft.gov.uk/applicants.php> (Accessed 7 September 2005).
54 Department of Health (2003), *A Short Guide to NHS Foundation Trusts*, London: The Stationery Office, p. 4.
55 *Health and Social Care (Community Health and Standards) Act 2003*, London: The Stationery Office, section 39.
56 Monitor, Independent Regulator of NHS Foundation Trusts (2004), *NHS Foundation Trusts: Report on Elections and Membership (August 2004)*, London: Monitor.
57 Department of Health, 'Maps of treatment centre locations, NHS & IS TC schemes – February 05', online at <http://www.dh.gov.uk/PolicyAndGuidance/Organisation Policy/SecondaryCare/TreatmentCentres/fs/en> (Accessed 1 June 2005).
58 NHS Modernisation Agency, 'Delivery and excellence in elective care', *Cutting Edge*, issue 3 (August 2004), p. 1.
59 Department of Health (December 2004), *Chief Executives Report to the NHS*, London: The Stationery Office, p. 11.
60 Milburn A., Secretary of State for Health (12 June 2002), *Empowering Front Line Staff*, speech to the British Association of Medical Managers (BAMMs) conference.

61 Laing and Buisson (2004), *Laing's Healthcare Market Review, 2004–2005*, p. 55, Table 2.1, p. 56.
62 Figures for 1997–98, the latest data available Laing and Buisson (2004), *Laing's Healthcare Market Review, 2004–2005*, Table 2.18, p. 110.
63 Laing and Buisson (2004), *Laing's Healthcare Market Review, 2004–2005*, Figure 2.4, p. 60.
64 Department of Health (2004), *Departmental Report 2004*, p. 57
65 Laing and Buisson (2004), *Laing's Healthcare Market Review, 2004–2005*, p. 62.
66 NHS Health and Social Care Information Centre, *HES [free data], table 4, main operations summary 2003–2004*, p. 4, online at <http://www.hesonline.nhs.uk/Ease/servlet/DynamicPageBuild?siteID=1802&categoryID=204&catName=Main%20operations:%20summary> (Accessed 7 June 2005).
67 Department of Health (2004), *The NHS Improvement Plan*, p. 52.
68 Department of Health (2005), *Creating a Patient Led NHS – Delivering the NHS Improvement Plan*, London: The Stationery Office, p. 21.
69 Laing and Buisson (2004), *Laing's Healthcare Market Review, 2004–2005*, Table 2.5, p. 69.
70 Ibid., pp. 74, 75.
71 Ibid., p. 70.
72 Ibid., p. 99.
73 Ibid., p. 97.
74 Ibid., p. 77.
75 Department of Health (2004), *Departmental Report 2004*, London: The Stationery Office, p. 58.
76 Department of Health (2002), *Treating More Patients and Extending Choice: Overseas Treatment for NHS Patients*, London: The Stationery Office, p. 12.
77 Reid J., Secretary of State for Health, in: Department of Health (2004), *The NHS Improvement Plan*, Preface, p. 7.
78 Faculty of Public Health Medicine (2003), *Statement on Managed Public Health Networks*, London: Faculty of Public Health Medicine.
79 London Health Observatory, 'Staff list for the London Health Observatory 2004', online at <http://www.lho.org.uk/Aboutus/Contact us.htm> (Accessed 4 November 2004).
80 Health Protection Agency (2004), *Summary of Corporate Plan, 2004–2009*, London: Health Protection Agency, p. 20.
81 Ibid.

5 Funding and resources

1 The United Kingdom Parliament, Hansard written answers for 1 March 2005, online at <http://www.parliament.the-stationery-office.co.uk/pa/cm200405/cmhansard/cm050301/text/50301w12.htm> (Accessed 3 September 2005).
2 HM Treasury, *2004 government spending review*, Chapter 8, Tables 8.1 and 8.2, p. 100, online at <http://www.hm-treasury.gov.uk/media//7C2D8/sr2004_ch8.pdf> (Accessed 13 June 2005).
3 Department of Health (2005), *Departmental Report 2005*, Chapter 3, p. 43, online at < http://www.dh.gov.uk/assetRoot/04/11/71/54/04117154.pdf> (Accessed 3 September 2005).
4 Ibid., Chapter 3, Figure 3.8, p. 40.
5 Department of Health (2004), *2004–2005 Primary Medical Services Allocations*, AWP(05–06)PCT15, Leeds: Department of Health, Annex K.
6 House of Commons Health Committee (2005), *Public Expenditure on Health and Personal Social Services 2004*, Table 3.1.3.

7 Department of Health (2004), *Report of the Primary Care Dental Workforce Review*, London: Department of Health, p. 5.

8 Department of Health (2004), *2005–2006 Primary Medical Services Allocation*, Annex B.

9 Department of Health (2003), *Investing in General Practice, the New General Medical Services Contract*, London: The Stationery Office, p. 39.

10 Ibid., p. 11.

11 Department of Health (2004), *Sustaining Innovation Through New PMS Arrangements*, London: The Stationery Office, p. 3.

12 British Medical Association, 'New GMS contract funding streams', online at <http://www.bma.org.uk/ap.nsf/content/fundingstreams> (Accessed 2 February 2005).

13 Department of Health (2003), *Investing in General Practice, the New General Medical Services Contract*, p. 20.

14 Royal College of General Practitioners (2004), *New GMS Contract (Overview and Resources Guide)*, London: Royal College of General Practitioners, 2004, p. 16, RCGP information sheet no. 6.

15 Department of Health (2005), *Primary Care Trust Recurrent Revenue Allocations 2006/07 and 2007/08*, Leeds: Department of Health, Health Services Circular 2005/001, p. 3.

16 Hudson, B. (2004), 'Policy into practice, partnership working between health and social care: the health act 1999', *Research, Policy and Planning*, vol. 22, no. 1, p. 57.

17 Department of Health in Wanless D. (2002), *Securing our Future Health: Taking a Long-term View*, London: HM Treasury, Final report, pp. 19, 32.

18 Department of Health (2003), *2003–2004 to 2005–2006 HCHS Capital Allocations*, Leeds: Department of Health, HSC2003/004, p. 1.

19 Department of Health, *New Delegated Limits for Capital Investment*, Leeds: Department of Health, 2003, p. 1.

20 Department of Health (2003), *2003–2004 to 2005–2006 HCHS Capital Allocations*, Annex C.

21 Ibid., p. 2.

22 Department of Health (2004), *Departmental Report 2004*, Chapter 4, pp. 49 and 51.

23 Department of Health (2003), *New Delegated Limits for Capital Investment*, p. 3 and Appendix 2.

24 Department of Health (2004), *Departmental Report 2004*, Chapter 4, pp. 51 and 52.

25 D. Gaffney and A. Pollock (1998), *Has the NHS Returned to Strategic Planning? The CPAG and the Second Wave of PFI*, London, Unison Health Care.

26 House of Commons Health Committee (2003), *Public Expenditure on Health and Personal Social Services 2001*, Questions 5.2.3 and 5.2.5.

27 Department of Health (2004), *2004–2005 Primary Medical Services Allocations*, Annex D.

28 Department of Health (2004), *National Health Service (General Medical Services – Premises Costs) Directions 2004*, London: The Stationery Office.

29 Department of Health (2004), *2004/2005 and 2005/2006 Primary Care Premises Funding*, Leeds, Annex.

30 Pollock A., Player S. and Godden S. (2001), 'How private finance is moving primary care into corporate ownership', *British Medical Journal*, 322: 960–3.

31 Department of Health (2000), *The NHS Plan: A Plan for Investment, a Plan for Reform*, p. 45.

32 Department of Health, 'About NHS LIFT', online, at <http://www.dh.gov.uk/procurementandproposals/publicprivatepartnerships/NHSLIFT/fs/en> (Accessed 16 February 2005).

33 Department of Health, 'Unified exposition book: 2003/2004, 2004/2005 & 2005/2006 PCT revenue resource limits', Table 3.4 other (CFISSA), online at <http://www.

dh.gov.uk/policyanduidance/organisationpolicy/financeanplanning/allocations/fs/en> (Accessed 16 February 2005).

34 Department of Health (2003) *The NHS Contractors Companion*, London: Department of Health.

35 Department of Health, *Payment by Results Core Tools 2004*, main document, p. 12, online at <http://www.dh.gov.uk/policyanduidance/organisationpolicy/financeanplanning/NHSfinancialreforms/NHSfinancialreformsarticle/fs/en?CONTENT_ID=4000333&chk=UzhHA3> (Accessed 16 February 2005).

36 Department of Health, *National Tariff 2005–2006*, Appendix A, online at <http://www.dh.gov.uk/policyanduidance/organisationpolicy/financeanplanning/NHSfinancialreforms/NHSfinancialreformsarticle/fs/en?CONTENT_ID=4091529&chk=f%2Bcvh8> (Accessed 16 February 2005).

37 Department of Health (2004), *The NHS Improvement Plan*, p. 29.

38 Department of Health (2002), *Delivering the NHS Plan. Next Steps on Investment, Next Steps on Reform*, London: The Stationery Office, pp. 8, 22–3.

39 Department of Health (2004), *Local Authority Circular 2004(3)*, London: The Stationery Office, p. 2, online at <http://www.dh.gov.uk/assetRoot/04/07/33/53/04073353.PDF> (Accessed 22 February 2005).

40 Department of Health (2004), *Departmental Report 2004*, Chapter 7, p. 105.

41 Department of Health (2005), *Departmental Report 2005*, Chapter 7, p. 119.

42 Department of Health, 'NHS financial manual, NHS trusts detailed guidance, 13 NHS trust financing', p. 12, online at http://www.info.doh.gov.uk/doh/finman.nsf/ManualDownload?OpenView (Accessed 16 January 2005).

43 Department of Health, 'Funding of strategic health authorities and primary care trusts', pp. 15–16, online at http://www.info.doh.gov.uk/doh/finman.nsf/ManualDownload?OpenView (Accessed 16 January 2005).

44 Department of Health (2002) *Delivering the NHS Plan. Next Steps on Investment, Next Steps on Reform*, p. 30.

45 Department of Health (2004), *Departmental Report 2004*, Chapter 7, p. 61.

6 Efficiency and standards

1 Department of Health (2000), *The NHS Plan: A Plan for Investment, a Plan for Reform*, London: The Stationery Office, Chapter 6, p. 59.

2 Department of Health (2002), *Improvement, Expansion and Reform, National Priorities and Planning Framework 2003/04–2005/06*, London: The Stationery Office, Appendix B.

3 Department of Health (2004), *National Standards Local Action, Health and Social Care Standards and Planning Framework, 2005/06–2007/08*, London: The Stationery Office, Annex B.

4 Ibid., pp. 28–34.

5 Department of Health, *Performance Assessment Framework of Strategic Health Authorities, The Framework and Assessment Questionnaire 2003/2004*, online at <http://www.dh.gov.uk/assetRoot/04/08/56/56/04085656.pdf> (Accessed 9 November 2004).

6 Department of Health (2004), *Reconfiguring the Department of Health's Arm's Length Bodies*, London: The Stationery Office, p. 35.

7 Independent Regulator of NHS Foundation Trusts, *Update on Bradford Teaching Hospitals NHS Foundation Trust*, 26/11/2004, online, at <http://www.monitor-nhsft.gov.uk/news.php?id=568> (Accessed 7 December 2005).

8 Department of Health (1999), *Clinical Governance. Quality in the New NHS*, HSC 1999/065, Leeds: Department of Health, Annex 2.

9 Department of Health (2004), Departmental report 2004, p. 59.

10 British Medical Association, 'New GMS contract funding streams', online at <http://www.bma.org.uk/ap.nsf/content/fundingstreams> (Accessed 2 February 2005).

11 General Medical Council, 'About us: protecting the public', online at <http://www.gmc-uk.org/about/default.htm> (Accessed 5 March 2005).

12 Council for Healthcare Regulatory Excellence, *Frequently Asked Questions about the Council for Healthcare Regulatory Excellence*, online at <http://www.chre.org.uk/Website/faq.doc> (Accessed 3 March 2005).

13 Chief Dental Officer (2004), *The National Clinical Assessment Authority – Here to Help*, CDO update September 2004, London: Department of Health.

14 Chief Medical Officer (2003), *Annual Report of the Chief Medical Officer 2002, Progress Made by the National Clinical Assessment Authority*, CMO update 36, London: Department of Health, p.2.

15 Department of Health (2004), *Reconfiguring the Department of Health's Arm's Length Bodies*, London: The Stationery Office, p. 22.

16 National Patient Safety Agency, 'Our work', online at <http://www.npsa.nhs.uk/npsa/work> (Accessed 5 March 2005).

17 Department of Health (2000), *The NHS Plan: A Plan for Investment, a Plan for Reform*, Chapter 10, pp. 88–95.

18 Department of Health (2004), *Reconfiguring the Department of Health's Arm's Length Bodies*, Annex B.

19 Commission for Patient and Public Involvement in Health (November 2004), *Forum Members' Handbook*, p. 4, online at <http://www.cppih.org/ppi_downloads.html> (Accessed 8 March 2005).

20 Commission for Patient and Public Involvement in Health (November 2004), *Forum Members' Handbook*, online at <http://www.cppih.org/ppi_downloads.html> (Accessed 8 March 2005).

21 Department of Health (2000), *The NHS Plan: A Plan for Investment, a Plan for Reform*, Chapter 10, pp. 91, 92.

22 Department of Health (2004), *Independent Complaints Advocacy Service (ICAS). The First Year of ICAS: 1 September 2003–31 August 2004*, London: The Stationery Office, pp. 4 and 7.

23 Department of Health, 'NHS written complaints data files available for download', online at <http://www.performance.doh.gov.uk/hospitalactivity/data_requests/nhs_complaints.htm> (Accessed 8 March 2005).

24 Department of Health, 'How to make a complaint about the NHS' online at <http://www.dh.gov.uk/PolicyAndGuidance/OrganisationPolicy/ComplaintsPolicy/NHSComplaintsProcdure/fs/en> (Accessed 8 March 2005).

25 *Statutory Instrument 2004 No. 1767, The National Health Service (Complaints) Regulations 2004*, London: The Stationery Office.

26 Department of Health (2003), *Making Amends. A Consultation Paper Setting out Proposals for Reforming the Approach to Clinical Negligence in the NHS. A Report by the Chief Medical Officer*, London: The Stationery Office, p. 106.

27 The NHS Litigation Authority, *About the NHS Litigation Authority*, online at <http://www.nhsla.com/home.htm> (Accessed 9 March 2005).

7 Research and development, and research governance

1 Department of Health, 'Research and development', online at <http://www.dh.gov.uk/PolicyAndGuidance/ResearchAndDevelopment/ResearchAndDevelopmentAZ/PrioritiesForResearch/fs/en?CONTENT_ID=4069152&chk=81UxOy> (Accessed 6 June 2005).

2 Department of Health (2000), *Research & Development for a First Class Service, R&D in the new NHS*, London: The Stationery Office.

3 Department of Health (2001), *Research Governance Framework for Health and Social Care*, London: The Stationery Office.
4 House of Lords Select Committee on Science and Technology (1988), *Priorities in Medical Research, Volume 1 – Report*, London: The Stationery Office.
5 Culyer, A. (1994), *Supporting Research and Development in the NHS, Report of the Department of Health Research and Development Task Force*, London: The Stationery Office.
6 Arnold, E., Morrow S., Thuriaux, B. and Martin, B. (1999) *Implementing the Culyer Reforms in North Thames: Final Report, Science and Technology Policy Research*, London, Technopolis. Black, N. (1997), 'A national strategy for research and development: lessons from England', *Annual Review of Public Health*, vol. 18, pp.485–505. Harrison, A. and New, B. (2001), 'The finance of research and development in health care', *Health Care UK*, pp. 26–44. Harrison, A. and New, B. (2002), *Public Interest, Private Decisions: Health-related Research in the UK*, London: King's Fund, within and p. 16.
7 Millar, B. (1998), 'R&D: Failing the acid test', *Health Service Journal*, 26 March, pp. 24–7.
8 Department of Health (1999), *Strategic Review of the NHS R&D Levy: Final Report*, London: Department of Health.
9 Her Majesty's Treasury, *Selling Government Services into Wider Markets, Policy and Guidance Note,* online at <http://www.hm-treasury.gov.uk/mediastore/otherfiles/sgswm.pdf> (Accessed 6 June 2005).
10 Department of Health (2000), *NHS R&D Funding Consultation Paper: NHS Support for Science*, London: The Stationery Office. Department of Health (2000), *NHS R&D Funding Consultation Paper: NHS Priorities and Needs Funding*, London: The Stationery Office. Department of Health (2001), *NHS Priorities and Needs R&D Funding: A Position Paper*, London: The Stationery Office.
11 Department of Health (2001), *Science and Innovation Strategy*, London: The Stationery Office, pp. 4 and 18.
12 Woods, K. (2004), Implementing the European clinical trials directive (editorial), *British Medical Journal* 328: 240–1.
13 Department of Health. Report of the ad hoc advisory group on the operation of NHS research ethics committees, London, 2005–08–26.
14 House of Commons Select Committee on Science and Technology (2000), *Cancer Research: A Fresh Look*, London: House of Commons.
15 National Cancer Research Institute (2002), *Strategic Analysis 2002: An Overview of Cancer Research in the UK Directly Funded by the NCRI Partner Organisations*, London: National Cancer Research Institute.
16 The Academy of Medical Sciences (2003), *Strengthening Clinical Research*, p. 7, online at <http://www.acmedsci.ac.uk/p_scr.pdf> (Accessed 6 June 2005).
17 Research for Patient Benefit Working Party, *Final report*, London, 2004, p. 1.
18 Office of Science and Technology (2001), *Public Sector Research Exploitation Fund – Basic Guidelines*, online at < http://www.ost.gov.uk/enterprise/knowledge/psrefundguide.pdf> (Accessed 6 June 2005).
19 Department of Health. Best Research for Best Health: A New National Health Research Strategy: The NHS contribution to health research in England: a consultation.
20 Harrison, A. and New, B. (2002) *Public Interest, Private Decisions: Health-Related Research in the UK*, London: Kings Fund.

8 The NHS workforce

1 Department of Health, *All Staff in the NHS, 1994 to 2004 (NHS Workforce)*, online at <http://www.dh.gov.uk/assetRoot/04/10/65/95/04106595.xls> (Accessed 6 June 2005).

2   Department of Health (2002), *Improvement, Expansion and Reform: The Next Three Years. Priorities and Planning Framework 2003–2006,* London: The Stationery Office, p. 23.

3   Department of Health (2004), *Delivering the NHS Improvement Plan: The Workforce Contribution,* London: The Stationery Office, p. 1.

4   Royal College of Nursing (2004), *Fragile future? A Review of the UK Nursing Labour Market in 2003,* London, p. 16.

5   Department of Health, *Hospital, Public Health and Community Health Service Medical and Dental Staff in England: 1994–2004,* Table 4, online at <http://www. dh.gov.uk/assetRoot/04/10/67/35/04106735.pdf> (Accessed 7 June 2005).

6   Organisation for Economic Co-operation and Development, 'Health data 2005 – country notes', online, available at <http://www.oecd.org/document/46/0,2340,en_ 2649_37407_34971438_1_1_1_37407,00.html> (Accessed 7 June 2005).

7   Department of Health (2004), *Sustaining Innovation Through New PMS Arrangements,* London: The Stationery Office, p. 3.

8   Department of Health (2005), *Statistics for General Medical Practitioners in England: 1994–2004,* pp. 2 and Table 1b, online at <www.dh.gov.uk/PublicationsandStatistics/ Statistics/StatisticalWorkAreas/Worforce/fs/en> (Accessed 20 April 2005).

9   Department of Health (2004), *NHS Dentistry: Delivering Change, a Report by the Chief Dental Officer (England),* London: The Stationery Office, p. 6.

10 Department of Health (2003), *Ophthalmic Statistics for England, 1993–94 to 2003–2004,* London: The Stationery Office, p. 1.

11 Department of Health (2004), *Departmental Report 2004,* p. 101.

12 Department of Health (2005), *NHS Hospital and Community Health Services Non-medical Staff in England, 1994–2004,* London: The Stationery Office, Tables 1b and 2b, online at <http://www.dh.gov.uk/assetRoot/04/10/67/31/04106731.pdf>

13 Unison, 'Healthcare', online at <http://www.unison.org.uk/healthcare/index.asp> (Accessed 20 August 2005).

14 Amicus, *Amicus and the health sector.* Amicus research, London, 2004, p. 11.

15 GMB, 'Healthcare sector', online at <http://www.gmb.org.uk/Templates/Internal. asp?NodeID=91299&int1stParentNodeID=89645&int2ndParentNodeID=89654&int 3rdParentNodeID=89986> (Accessed 26 August 2005).

16 British Medical Association, 'About the BMA', online at <http://www.bma.org.uk/ ap.nsf/Content/Hubaboutthebma> (Accessed 20 August, 2005).

9 Devolution

1   Dixon, J. and Klein, R. (1999), 'Is the English NHS underfunded?', *British Medical Journal,* vol. 318: 522–6.

2   Office for National Statistics, 'Population estimates', online at <http://www.statistics. gov.uk/cci/nugget.asp?id=6> (Accessed 15 March 2005).

3   Scottish Executive Health Department, 'About us', online, at <http://www.show.scot. nhs.uk/sehd/about.htm> (Accessed 15 March 2005).

4   Scottish Intercollegiate Guidelines Network, 'What is SIGN?', online at <http://www. sign.ac.uk/about/introduction.html> (Accessed 17 March 2005).

5   NHS Wales, Directly Employed NHS Staff in Post at 30 September 2003, Table A 14.10, online at <http://www.wales.gov.uk/keypubstatisticsforwales/content/ publication/health/2004/hsw2005/hsw2005-ch14/hsw2005-ta14-10.xls> (Accessed 5 April 2005).

6   NHS Wales, 'What is NHS Wales?' online at <http://www.wales.nhs.uk/page. cfm?pid=3331> (Accessed 5 April 2005).

7   Department of Health, Social Services, and Public Safety (2002), *Health and Social Care in Northern Ireland, a Statistical Profile,* Northern Ireland: Department of Health, Social Services, and Public Safety, p. 8.

8 Department of Health, Social Services, and Public Safety, *Health and Personal Social Services Workforce: 1994–2003*, online at <http://www.dhsspsni.gov.uk/publications/2004/workcensus/TableA.pdf> (Accessed 22 March 2005).
9 Department of Health, Social Services and Public Safety (2003), *Local Health and Social Care Groups*, p. 1, online at <http://www.n-i.nhs.uk/lhascg/LHASCG.pdf> (Accessed 7 December 2005).
10 Department of Health, Social Services and Public Safety (2004), *A Healthier Future: A 20 year Vision for Health and Well-being in Northern Ireland, 2005–2025*, Northern Ireland: Department of Health, Social Services, and Public Safety.

10 The future

1 Secretary of State for Health, *Our Health, Our Care, Our Say: A New Direction for Community Services*, Cm. 6737, January 2006.
2 UnitedHealth Europe are to provide general practice services in Derbyshire, and Central Surrey Health, a co-ownership company, will provide nursing and other services to Mid Surrey PCT (*Guardian*, Friday 13 January 2006), online at <http://society.guardian.co.uk/health/story/0,,1693738,00.html>.
3 Ibid.
4 Seamus Ward, 'A shot in the arm', *Public Finance*, 7 October 2005; John Carvel, 'Hit squads to tackle £900m NHS deficit', *Guardian,* 2 December 2005.
5 'Surgery delayed and patients removed from waiting lists to save money', *The Times*, 3 December 2005; 'North Staffordshire's PCTs are planning to withdraw £130,000 annually from a pioneering walk-in centre at Burslem's Haywood Hospital as they struggle to claw back millions of pounds of debt. This would leave the Haywood centre with just its £800,000 of central government funding, undermining its ability to hit the four-hour waiting target. This week Newcastle PCT also announced it will be pulling funding from cancer services and a mental health care initiative', *Stoke Sentinel*, http://www.thisisthesentinel.co.uk.
6 'Hospital trust attacked for taking heart patients off list', *Financial Times*, 3 January 2006.
7 'Two-tier NHS care for pregnant women ready to pay £4,000. The Queen Charlotte's and Chelsea Hospital, London, is offering pregnant women higher quality maternity care for £4,000. The service includes home visits by a midwife, 24-hour telephone contact, pre-natal classes including a birth rehearsal and one-on-one care in the later stages of pregnancy. The Royal College of Midwives and the Royal College of Nursing have expressed deep concern about the scheme, which is only available to women who can pay', online at <http://www.telegraph.co.uk/news/main.jhtml ?xml=/news/2006/01/21/nhs21.xml>.
   'NHS hospital charging for private MRI scans. The Royal Cornwall Hospital in Truro offers MRI scans to fee-paying private customers, whilst there is reportedly an 11-month waiting list for NHS patients who need to use the facility. The hospital claims it needs the money from private treatment to subsidise the cost of NHS scans. Lack of funding has meant the scanner has been underused since it was installed in September. Now the hospital has slashed the fee to private patients in a bid to attract more custom. It has denied it is involved in a price war with other NHS centres', online at <http://news.bbc.co.uk/1/hi/england/cornwall/4666146.stm>.
8 UnitedHealth, the global healthcare corporation mentioned previously, are no strangers to fraud: 'Travelers, UnitedHealth settle Medicare fraud lawsuit for $20.6 million', California Healthline, 13 August 2004, online at <http://www.californiahealthline.org/index.cfm?Action=dspItem&itemID=104917&ClassCD=CL113>. Another major Health Maintenance Organisation, Columbia-HCA, made an agreed settlement of $745 million with the US Department of Justice in 2000 for fraud and abuse of the Medicare programme. In the same year Columbia-HCA owned the fourth largest

number of private hospitals in the UK. The FBI estimated the value of healthcare fraud in the USA from 1990 to 1995 at no less than \$418 billion (*Health Care – Private Corporations or Public Service? The Americanisation of the NHS*, third report of the Health Policy Network, London 1996, pp. 29–32).

9 The most publicized was Ms. Hewitt's recall of an imminent PFI scheme for St Bartholomew's and the Royal London hospitals in London, but there were others, giving rise to a widespread feeling that the future of the PFI was now in doubt. For example: 'PFI doubts lead Hewitt to turn down hospital's trust application'. 'An application by the University Hospitals of Leicester trust has been put on hold while its £761m PFI scheme is reviewed. There are rumours in the PFI market that there is a six month moratorium on new PFI hospitals, something the Department of Health denies', *Financial Times*, 19 January 2006; 'Cash crisis threatens plans for more PFI hospitals ... Two more hospital PFI schemes have been held up by fears over affordability – the Plymouth Hospitals Vanguard PFI project, with a value of £600m, and the Hillingdon Hospital in Uxbridge, West London, a £300m scheme. In the case of Plymouth, officials are questioning whether a proposed £200m care centre will be able to compete with enhanced GP surgeries and IS-TCs', *The Times*, 18 January 2006, online at <http://www.timesonline.co.uk/article/0,,2-1990917,00.html>.

10 Steffie Woolhandler, Terry Campbell, and David Himmelstein, 'Costs of health care administration in the United States and Canada', *The New England Journal of Medicine*, 23 January 2003; Steffie Woolhandler and David Himmelstein, 'Taking care of business: HMOs that spend more on administration deliver lower quality care', *International Journal of Health Services*, Vol. 32, 2002. According to Woolhandler and Himmelstein, in a comparison between administrative costs in the US and Canada, 'After exclusions administration accounted for 31% of health care expenditures in the US and 16.7% of health care expenditures in Canada'. See also P.J. Deverau, P.T.L. Choi, C. Lachette, *et al.*, 'A systematic review of and meta-analysis of studies comparing mortality rates of private for-profit and not-for-profit hospitals', *CMAJ*, Vol. 166, 2002. A recent estimate put the US figure for administrative costs at 25% of healthcare spending: see James G. Kahn, Richard Kronick, Mary Kreger and David N Gans, 'The cost of health insurance administration in California: estimates for insurers, physicians and hospitals', *Health Affairs*, Vol. 24, January/February 2006.

Index

national standards 104–7, 110–11, *see also* standards
national targets 109–10, 118–19
national tariff 9, 40, 97–8
National Workforce Group 147
nationally directed services 53–4
nationally enhanced services 54
NatPaCT 125
NCAS 122–3, 163
NCRI 143
NCRN 143
NEAT 140
need for healthcare services: in devolved countries 155, 159; and distribution of revenue 4–5; and provision by FTs 112–13; within a market-based system 9–10
negligence, clinical 25–6, 132, 134–5
NES 158
networks: for clinical research 143–5; public health 36, 62, 73–4, 168; for Scottish primary medical service 159–60
The New NHS: Modern, Dependable 132
NHS: accountability of 127; expenditure as per cent of GDP and compared with other countries 78–9; from 1911–1980 2–5; government funding of 2–3, 78–9; the new market 7–10; in Northern Ireland 169–76, 177; private funding of 2, 68, 78; role and structure of 3–10, 157–9, 164–9, 170–6; in Scotland 157–64, 177; transition to market-based system 1, 5–7, 104–7; in Wales 164–9
NHS 24 158, 159
NHS Appointments Commission 31–2, 127, 128, 129
NHS Bank 103
NHS BT 29–30
NHS and Community Care Act 1990 6, 61, 137
NHS Complaints Reform – Making Things Right 132
NHS Counter Fraud and Security Management Service 25
NHS Direct 49, 53–4
NHS Education Scotland 163
NHS Employers 14
NHS estate *see* estate
NHS executive, before 1980 5
NHS Gateway to Leadership Programme 153
NHS Health Scotland 158
NHS ILSI 24–5, 124–6, 125

NHS Indemnity 134
NHS Information Authority 27
NHS LIFT 41, 94–5
NHS Modernisation Board 17–18
NHS Pensions Agency 25
The NHS Plan (2000): care trusts 44; funding and resources 89–90; national targets set 109; NHS and independent sector 68; NHS Modernisation Board 17–18; patient–public involvement 127; performance assessment 117; privatization 7; regulatory councils 122; research and development 136; workforce development 147, 152
NHS R&D levy 137, 139
NHS Redress Scheme 135
NHS Reform and Healthcare Professions Act 2002 122, 127, 164, 169
NHS Reform (Scotland) Act 2004 157
NHS Scotland 157–64, 177
NHS trusts: accountability of 111–13; capital charges 100; contracts 6, 40, 62, 97; cost of services 96; financial duties of 101–2; function and structure of 61–3; and independent sector 62–3; lay representation on boards 127–8, 163, 169; national targets for 109, 110; in Northern Ireland 173, 175, 176; operating surpluses 90; and payment by results 97; performance assessment 111–12; performance management 108; private facilities 70; private patient income 62; provision of community health services 59–60; and research governance 141; resource allocations 61–3; sale of assets 61–2, 90; in Wales 167, 168, 169, *see also* care trusts; FTs; PCTs
NHS University 24, 125–6
NHS Wales 164–9
NHS (Wales) Act 2003 169
NHSLA 25–7, 134–5
NHSWD 164–6
NICE 28–9, 75, 113–14, 140, 162, 175
NIMHE 125
non-clinical services, outsourcing 5
non-clinical staff *see* non-medical staff
non-consultant career grades 123, 150
non-DH funding sources, for PCTs 87
non-discretionary funding 80, 82
non-executive members: of NHS boards 127–8, 130; of Northern Ireland boards 176; of PCT boards 42; of Scottish boards 163

non-medical staff 126–7, 153–4, 163;
    numbers of, in NHS 148
non-NHS bodies, becoming FTs 64
non-training posts 150
Northern Ireland 156, 169–76, 177
Northern Ireland Adverse Incident Centre
    176
notional rent 92
NPfIT 23, 90, 110, 125, *see also*
    information
NPSA 27–8, 122–3, 124, 126, 169, 176
NRLS 126
NSFs 10, 113, 114, 140, 162, 168
NTA 29
NTRAC 143
nurse consultants 147, 152
nurse-led: community care services 39,
    59–60; primary care services 52–3
Nursing and Midwifery Council 151
nursing staff 151–2; numbers of, in NHS
    148; primary care role 49, *see also*
    staff; workforce

Ombudsman, Health Service 134
one stop shop 93, 94
online appointments' booking 23
operating divisions, of HPA 159, 160
operating surpluses 90
operational capital 88–9
ophthalmic services, NHS 57, 82, 151
organ donation services 29–30
An Organisation with a Memory 126
Our Health, Our Care (DH publication) 178
Our National Health (NHS Scotland) 157
out of hours services: GP services 38–9,
    51, 85; NHS 24 158, 159; NHS Direct
    49, 53–4
outcomes: quality and outcomes
    framework 86–7, 121; targets for 109
outsourcing (contracting out) 5
overseas medical staff 67, 148–9
overseas patients 62, 71
overseas treatment providers 71
Overview and Scrutiny Committees 118,
    127, 131–2

pace of change 85, 89
PALS 127, 130
Parliament: accountability to 104; annual
    audit arrangements 102; ministerial
    responsibility 12, 13; Monitor
    accountable to 31
partnerships: care trusts 44–6; ChTs 47;
    in clinical research 142–5; FTs 64;

GPs 151; NHS and private sector
    70–1; in Northern Ireland 173; PCTs
    and local authorities 36, 38, 62, 87;
    PCTs and other NHS bodies 62; in
    public health 73–4; public–private
    70–1, 94–5, 100, 139, 144–5; Scottish
    community health 160, 163; Welsh
    LHBs 166–7, 168, 169
Partnerships for Care 157
Partnerships for Health 94–5
PASA 21–3, 25
pathfinder ChTs 46
patient access *see* access
patient choice *see* choice
patient constituency, of FTs 65, 128
patient discharge 99–100
patient pathways 160
patient prospectuses 132
patient–public involvement 4; in Northern
    Ireland 176; and performance
    management 107; PPI forums 32,
    42, 129–30, 163; in Scotland 163–4;
    standards for 114–16, 127–32; in
    Wales 169
patients: private 62, 68, 69–70;
    supplementary funding by 180
pay structures: Agenda for Change 10,
    126, 163, 176; of GPs 52; of hospital
    doctors 151, 177; of non-medical staff
    126–7, 163, *see also* contracts
Paymaster General 103
payment by results 9, 96–9, 156, 176, 179
payments and prices 25; for dental
    services 56; electronic system for 23;
    of GP practices 51–2; for independent
    sector services 99; for prescriptions
    25, 57–8
payments and prices public sector policy
    100
PCT MS 39, 50
PCTs (Primary Care Trusts):
    accountability of 111–12; additional
    income 87; capital allocation and
    distribution 93; capital charges
    100; changing role of 40, 41, 43–4;
    commissioning 7, 36–41, 53–4, 62,
    69, 178; financial duties of 101;
    foundation status of 41; and FTS 64;
    and general ophthalmic services 57;
    and GP practice-based commissioning
    43–4, 62; lay representation on boards
    127–8; national targets for 109, 110;
    and NHS dentistry 55–6; and NHS
    pharma services 58; partnerships

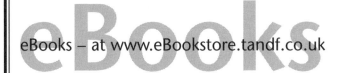